JAYLEE ALEXANDER

EXERCISE PROGRAMS FOR WOMEN

Empowering Women Through Fitness (2024 Guide for Beginners)

Copyright © 2023 by Jaylee Alexander

All rights reserved. No part of this publication may be reproduced, stored or transmitted in any form or by any means, electronic, mechanical, photocopying, recording, scanning, or otherwise without written permission from the publisher. It is illegal to copy this book, post it to a website, or distribute it by any other means without permission.

First edition

*This book was professionally typeset on Reedsy.
Find out more at reedsy.com*

Contents

1 Strength Training's Advantages for Women   1
2 Exercises for Strengthening at Home   4
3 Nutrition for Bodybuilders: What to Eat   21
4 Recipes for Clean Eating   25
5 Beginner's Guide to Strength Training   44
6 Beginner's Yoga   48
7 Beginner's Two-Week Yoga Training Plan: 55
8 Beginner's Two-Week Yoga Training Plan: Week Two   65
9 Advice for Newbies to Yoga   73

1

Strength Training's Advantages for Women

Most people assume strength training is only a male activity. The idea of bodybuilding was often derided by women who were afraid of coming across as "overly masculine." Rather, a lot of women have a tendency to devote a lot of time to various forms of training, such cardiovascular and mild toning activities. You can tone your muscles and lose body fat with these workouts, but until you start strength training, you won't be able to completely alter your body's shape.

Strength Training in the Pursuit of Loss of Weight

Every woman aspires to reduce her body fat and achieve the "hourglass shape." You must learn how to tone your core muscles and engage in cardio exercise if you want this amazing body. Your upper body will appear more defined as a result of strength training, which will increase the muscle in your back and shoulders. Strength training also draws attention to your hips and legs and provides your lower body that extra flare that makes you look more curvy. Women who lament their slender arms may find that their biceps and triceps need to be trained to address this issue.

Strength exercise, even for beginners, burns fat and calories. Your body goes through a sequence of resistance training exercises while you lift weights in order to gain muscle. This kind of workout raises your metabolism in addition to replacing fat with muscle. Your body starts burning calories day and night even while you are at rest when your resting metabolism rises. When it comes to weight loss, this is really beneficial. Gaining muscle entails increasing your calorie burn and reducing the fat deposits that have been bothering you with previous exercise regimens. You will become stronger and more slender after strength training.

Strength Training for Medical Purposes

Strength training for women also lowers the risk of osteoporosis, among other advantages. Lifting weights helps to build stronger bones in addition to stronger muscles. It lowers the risk of fractures and broken bones by increasing bone density. Weight training may be able to improve spinal bone density, giving you a stronger and healthier spine, according to research.

Strength training also lessens back pain and helps with posture. Weight training helps you acquire a taller physique with a straight spine, shoulders, and back by strengthening your core, back, and shoulders. It also helps you address improper posture. Additionally, it helps to avoid lower back problems.

Strength exercise improves your mood and lowers stress. Endorphins are released during exercise and weight training. These chemicals, called endorphins, combat melancholy, stop pain, and elevate mood in general. By stimulating the mind, an increase in endorphins also increases energy and enhances attentiveness.

Exercise to Increase Strength

Strength training can help you become more physically fit, avoid injuries, and perform other everyday chores like lifting and moving objects much more easily. It's possible that your hesitation to start strength training stems from your concern about appearing like the Incredible Hulk. Remain calm. Men experience all of that mass more often than women because hormones function differently in each gender. You can work out every day and add weight to your routine as a woman, but you'll never develop the massive biceps that you see on bodybuilders. Instead, you'll have a sleek, feminine style that is molded. Take note of every muscle in your body to build a robust, well-proportioned body.

The advantages of strength training are immense for females, so if you're not feeling motivated to pick up weights just yet, give it some serious thought. Give the at-home strength training exercises in this book a try, and you'll soon start to feel and look better.

2

Exercises for Strengthening at Home

Even while many bodybuilders like working out at gyms, if you're just starting out, you could feel more at ease at home. It's possible to perform numerous excellent weightlifting workouts in the comfort of your own house without the need for costly equipment or a specially designed gym. To get a sense of the types of movements and lifts you'll need to do to build strength, try these strength training exercises at home.

Exercises for Warm-Up

Starting a strength training program with a warm-up is crucial because it tells your body and mind that you will soon be engaging in some physical activity. These are a few crucial steps in preparing your body for more strenuous activity.

Heart

Warm up your heart for fifteen to twenty minutes. Your heart rate will increase, your metabolism will speed up, and your muscles will become relaxed and heated as a result. You should select the cardio option that appeals to you the most out of the various possibilities for your warm-up. You can increase the speed by jogging or even sprinting after your fast ten-minute walk. Ride a bike, jump rope, do some Zumba, or perform some aerobics. In order to proceed into the meat of your weight training program, the objective is to get your heart rate up and your body moving.

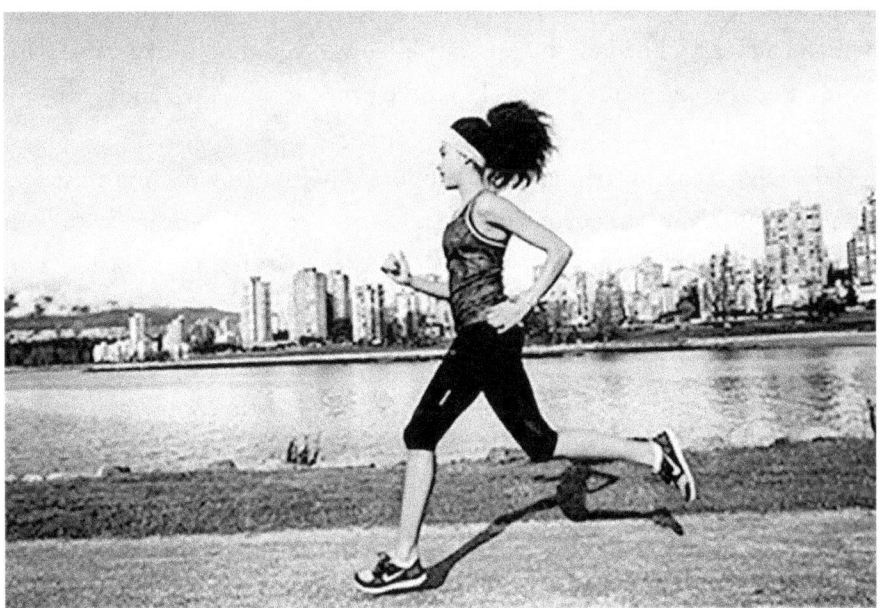

<u>Dynamic Extension</u>

A little adaptability will make a big difference. Your body will feel more flexible and you'll be able to move more effectively as you continue to tone it. Stretching will improve your flexibility and help you reach your strength objectives. Do it both before and after your workouts.

1. Begin with a few simple toe touches. Stretch your arms above your head while standing with your feet together and bending slightly at the waist. Even though there will be a tug at the back of your legs, keep lowering yourself to the ground. Aim to place the tips of your fingers on your toes. It's okay if you can't progress that far the first time. The harder you work at it, the closer you'll get. Reposition yourself to a standing position after a little while. Repeat five times.

2. Proceed to Linear Marches and Skips after that. The march is a basic

exercise in which you place your foot back on the ground after raising your knee to your waist. Carry out the same action using the opposite foot. March back and forth across your room three times. Next, turn it into a skip in which you leap while kicking up your knee and walking. Make sure to lift your knees to your waist as you skip three times around the room.

3. The next area to warm up is the upper body. Start by placing your feet shoulder-width apart, then perform a few arm circles. Beginning with your hands at your sides, raise both arms and execute a full circle with them. Perform ten swings in a forward motion and ten swings in a reverse direction.

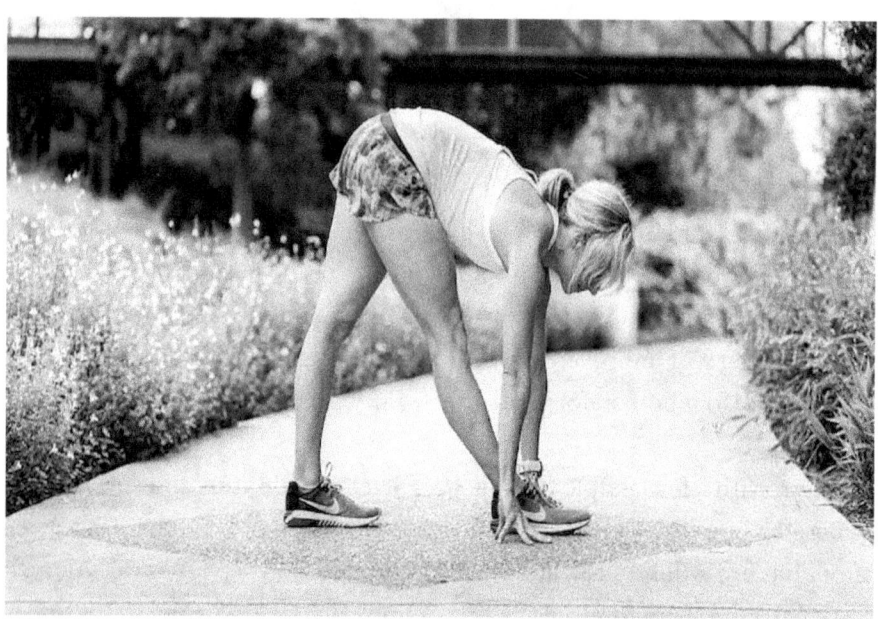

Harmony

Bodybuilding relies heavily on balance, thus learning how to maintain attention and balance your body weight should be part of your warm-up.

1. Before you dead lift, warm up. Place your feet together and keep your arms

by your sides as you stand. Raise your right arm and left leg together, then return both to the starting position. After ten repetitions, switch up and raise your left arm and right leg. Repeat those ten times as well.

2. Take a Duck Walk. Maintain a straight back as you squat and begin walking gently, never rising to a standing position but always staying in a squat. Go around your room three times in this manner.

3. Include some yoga. Lift your arms above your head while keeping your legs together. Raise your right leg and extend it ahead of you for a duration of ten seconds. Lower it and extend your left leg in the same manner. Finish five lifts on each leg.

Exercises for the Upper Body

When it comes to building your upper body, your back, shoulders, chest, and arms should be your main areas of concentration. These exercises can help you develop a stronger upper body and are simple enough for beginners to master. Basically, working the upper body involves pulling and pushing. These exercises are split into those two categories.

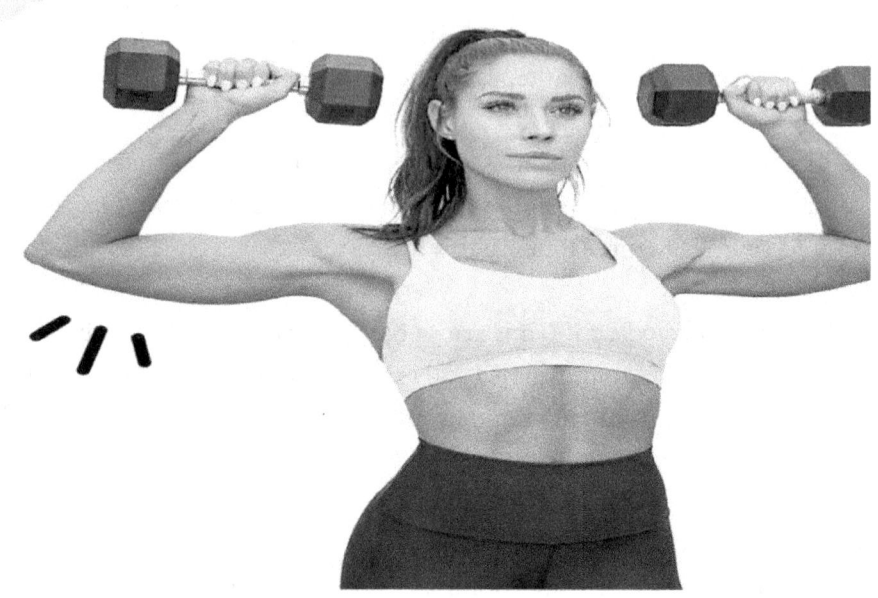

Pulling

1. Perform 12 dumbbell curls on each side in three sets. Choose a dumbbell weight that is comfortable for you to begin with. It may weigh three pounds, five pounds, or ten pounds. Use a bench or a chair for this workout. Lay your back flat and place one hand on the bench or chair's seat. Hold the dumbbell with your other hand while keeping your arm hanging straight at your side. When your elbow is parallel to the side of your body, bend and raise your arm. After a brief moment of holding, extend the arm once more.

2. Perform 12 dumbbell curls in 3 sets. Place a dumbbell in each hand and keep your arms straight while standing with your feet shoulder-width apart. Curl both of your arms up in front of you while bending them at the elbows. Hold for a moment before straightening them out once more.

3. Perform three sets of 12 weight pulls using a resistance stretch band. Step on the stretch band while holding onto both ends with your hands. In the

same manner as you did with the dumbbells, keep your arms straight and bend them to curl up.

Pressing

1. Place your palms flat on the ground in front of you, shoulder-width apart, while kneeling on the ground. Staying on your knees, descend your upper body toward the ground while maintaining a straight back. Push yourself back up as soon as you're almost touching your chin to the floor. As you gain strength, raise yourself off the ground and perform standard push-ups without contacting your knees.

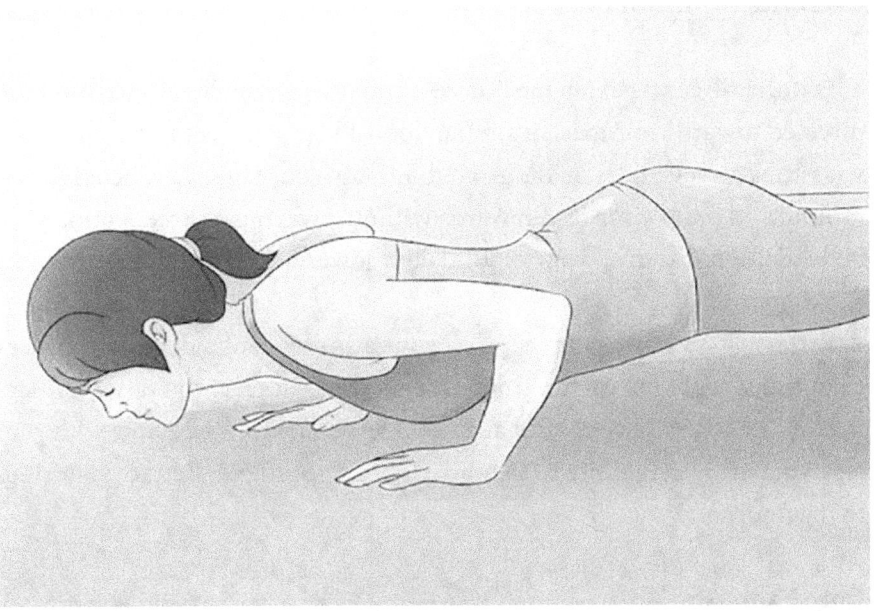

2. Perform 12 Trice Extensions in 3 Sets. With your arms bent and dumbbells in your hands, lie on your back. Raise and move the dumbbells away from your body until your arms reach nearly full length. Repeat by lowering them back to your chest. As much as possible, keep your elbows close to your torso.

3. Perform 12 shoulder extensions in 3 sets. Hold the dumbbells in your hands and stand with your legs shoulder-width apart. To position the weights at your shoulders, bend your arms. Raise them above your head and push them up until your arms are nearly straight. Return them to your shoulders slowly.

Workouts for the Core and Abs

Without a strong core, it is impossible to successfully construct your physique. Your lower back, glutes, and abs are all part of your core. These workouts will provide you with the fundamental strength needed to improve your bodybuilding outcomes.

Exercises for the Abdomen

1. Perform three sets of ten hip lifts. With your legs straight up and your head directed toward your toes, lie on the floor. Plant your feet firmly and keep your arms by your sides on the ground. Elevate your hips a few inches off the ground and point your feet upwards without swaying or accelerating your body. Once more, drop your hips till your lower back touches the ground.

2. Perform 10 V-Ups in 3 sets. With your arms by your sides and your legs extended straight out on the ground, lie on your back. As you raise your legs into a V stance, raise your head and shoulders concurrently. Along with your legs, your arms should rise so they are also off the ground. Retrace your steps to the floor.

Core Exercises

Perform 10 repetitions of the downward dog kick in 3 sets. Assume an inverted V position by pressing your hips up and back while on all fours. Raise your right leg and maintain a straight kick behind you. After ten reps, move to the left leg for ten more.

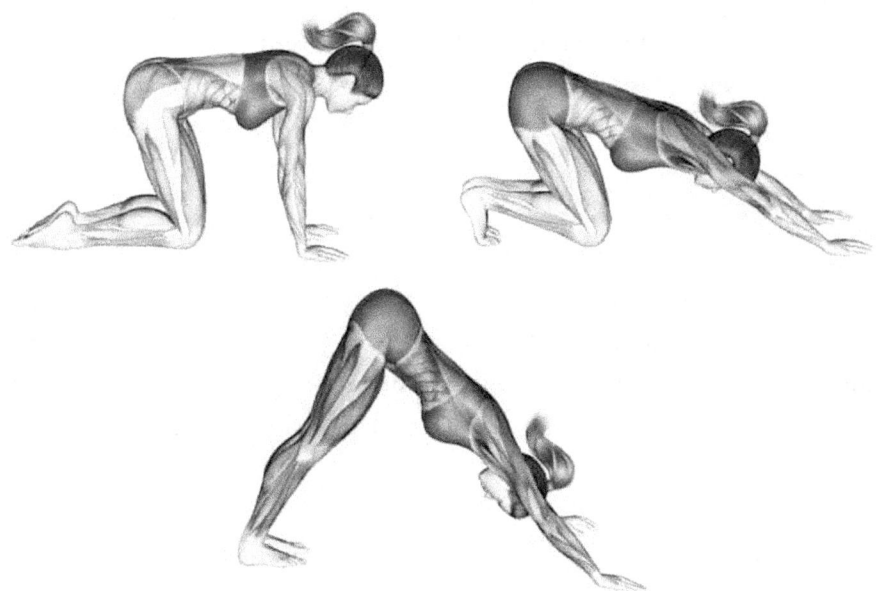

2. For a minimum of ten seconds, hold a plank three times. Lie flat on your stomach, with your hands flat on the ground, your elbows bent, and your toes curled beneath your feet. Assume the plank position by pushing yourself up until your back is flat and your arms are nearly straight (avoid locking the elbows). It is also possible to maintain this position with your elbows on the floor, however this is more challenging for most people.

Exercises for the Glutei

1. Perform 16 hip thrusts in three sets. With your knees bent and spaced shoulder-width apart, lie on your back. Maintaining your shoulders on the ground, push your hips toward the ceiling. After three seconds of holding the pose, return to the floor.

2. Perform 10 leg kicks in 3 sets. Place your hands and knees shoulder-width apart while on all fours. Raise your right leg as high as you can behind you while extending it straight. Without letting it make contact with the ground, bend and return the knee. Again, kick. After the right leg, kick the left.

Exercises for the Lower Body

You want to strengthen your hamstrings, quadriceps, hips, and thighs when working on your lower body. These workouts will improve range of motion, balance, and muscle growth.

Squats

1. Perform 12 squats in 3 sets. Place your hands on your hips and your legs shoulder-width apart as you stand. With your legs bent, carefully lower your torso toward the ground while maintaining a straight back. As low as you can go and still be able to push yourself back up to a standing position is the goal.

2. Perform three sets of ten weighted squats. With both hands, hold a dumbbell or kettlebell in front of you. Bend your arms and bring the weight up to your chest as you squat. As you straighten out of the squat, decrease the weight.

EXERCISES FOR STRENGTHENING AT HOME

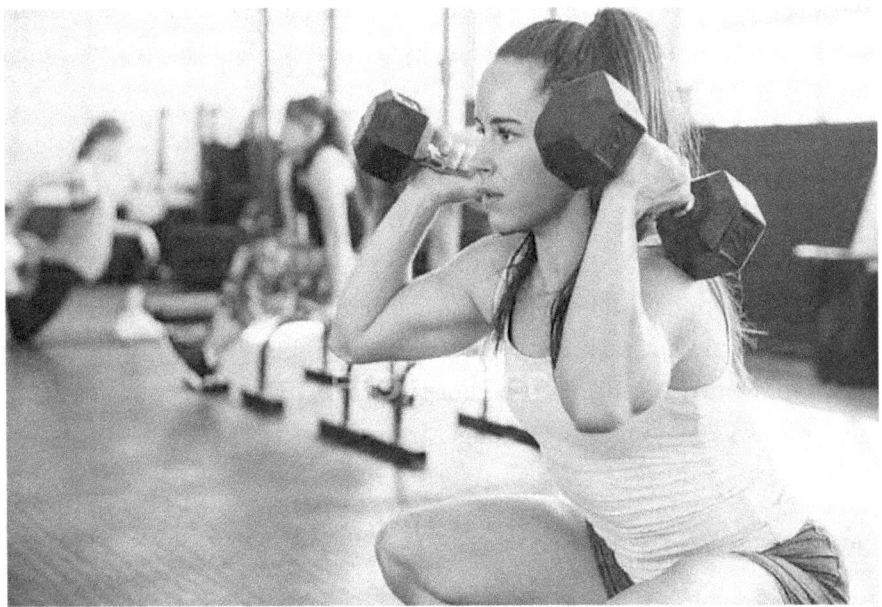

Lunges

1. Perform three sets of ten lunge steps. Step one forward while keeping your feet together, bending both legs until your back knee almost touches the ground and your leading leg reaches about 90 degrees. Maintain a straight back. Switch between your left and right leg.

2. Perform three sets of ten weighted lunge steps. With both hands, hold a single kettlebell or two dumbbells. As you bring the weights in front of you up to chest level, finish your lunges.

Jacks that Jump

The majority of us have performed jumping jacks at some point in our childhood. This exercise is excellent for strengthening the quadriceps, glutes, and hip flexors. As stabilizing muscles, it also works the shoulders, hamstrings, calves, and abs.

It is an excellent workout that increases both strength and endurance. Proceed to perform three sets of forty jumping jacks. This is a fantastic way to round off your day training.

Extra Lower Body Exercises

1. Perform ten hip abductions in three sets. Holding the back of a chair or a barre for support, stand with your legs together. While maintaining an upright and straight back, swing your right leg out to the side. Bring it back down to the floor. Repeat 10 on your right side, then move to your left leg. Your hips will get longer and stronger from this exercise.

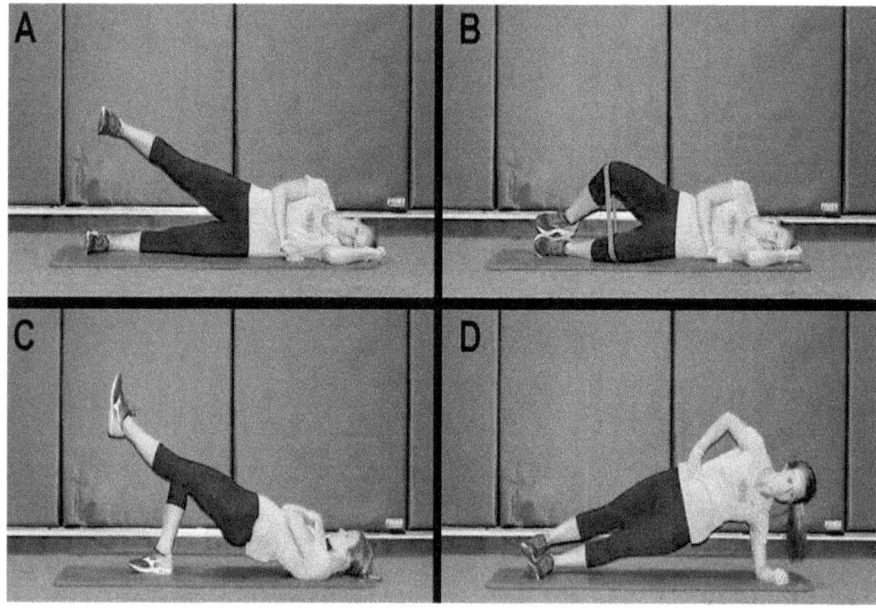

2. Perform 10 Hip Extenders in 3 sets. Holding the back of a chair or a barre for support, stand with your legs together. Maintaining a straight back and left leg, swing your right leg back behind you. Bring it back down to the floor. Repeat 10 on your right side, then move to your left leg.

3. Perform 15 toe raises in 3 sets. As you stand with your legs together, brace yourself with the back of a chair or a barre. Feel the muscles in your calves tense as you raise yourself up onto your toes. Return to the ground by lowering yourself. Take only a little break before pushing yourself back up onto your toes.

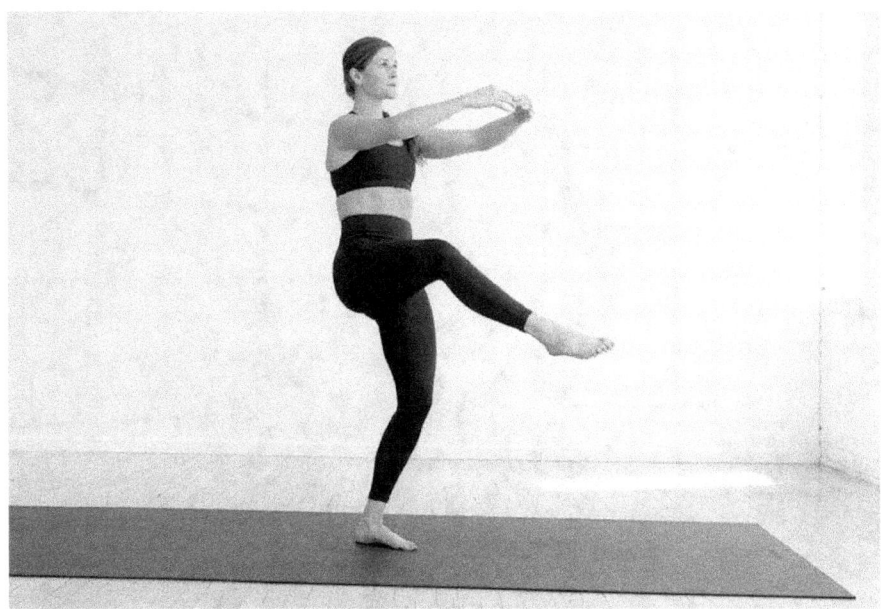

A Sample Training Schedule for Seven Days

You should plan your fitness regimen for several weeks at a time now that you know what kinds of workouts you may combine with at-home strength training activities. Make sure you are considering every aspect of strength training when you are making your plans. Resting is also necessary to allow your body and muscles to heal. This is an example of a 7-Day plan that would be a great starting point for bodybuilders.

Day 1: Lower Body

1. Warm up for ten minutes first. Take brisk walks around your area, or if you own a treadmill at home, use it. Since today is a lower body workout,

take an additional five minutes to warm up your hips and legs. Perform three marches and three skip sets.

2. Perform 12 squats in 3 sets.

3. Perform three sets of ten lunge steps.

4. Perform ten hip abductions on each leg in three sets.

5. Perform 3 sets of 10 leg-by-leg hip extenders.

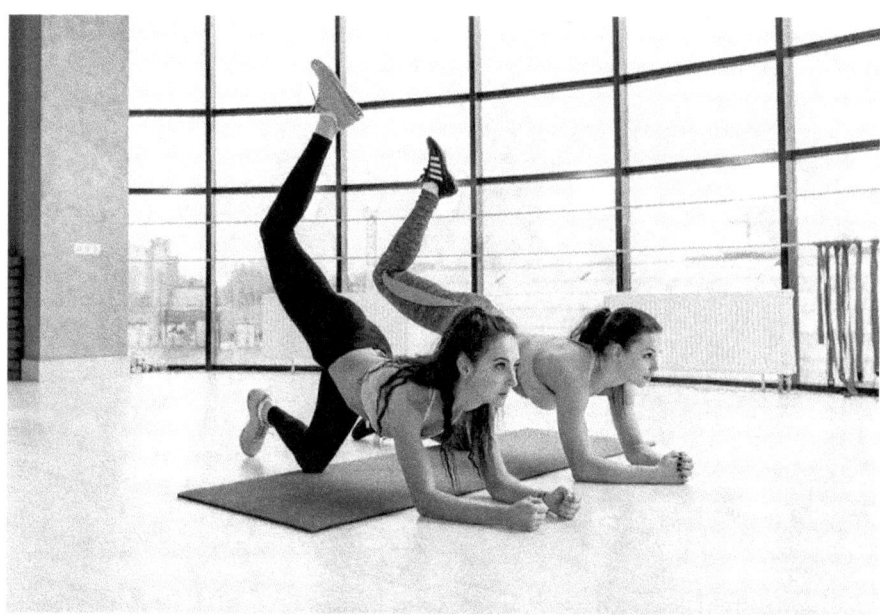

6. Assume a warrior posture. This yoga stance helps to strengthen the legs and lower back. Place your right foot, toe pointing forward, at least three or four feet in front of you. To maintain your balance and stretch your left leg as needed, turn it. Raise your arms over your head and fix your gaze on your palms, letting your front leg bear the majority of your weight. After at least 15 seconds of holding still, rotate such that your left leg is in front.

Day 2: Upper Body

1. Warm up for ten minutes first. Jog or stroll. Do three sets of ten arm circles to warm up your arms for an additional five minutes.

EXERCISES FOR STRENGTHENING AT HOME

2. Perform 10 push-ups in 3 sets.

3. Use a stretch band to perform three sets of 12 resistance pulls.

4. Perform 12 arm raises in 3 sets. With each hand, grasp a dumbbell, and maintain a straight arm position at your sides. Raise your arms above your head and maintain that position. Return them to rest by lowering them gradually. Raise them once more. Maintain a straight arm position.

5. Perform three more sets of ten push-ups.

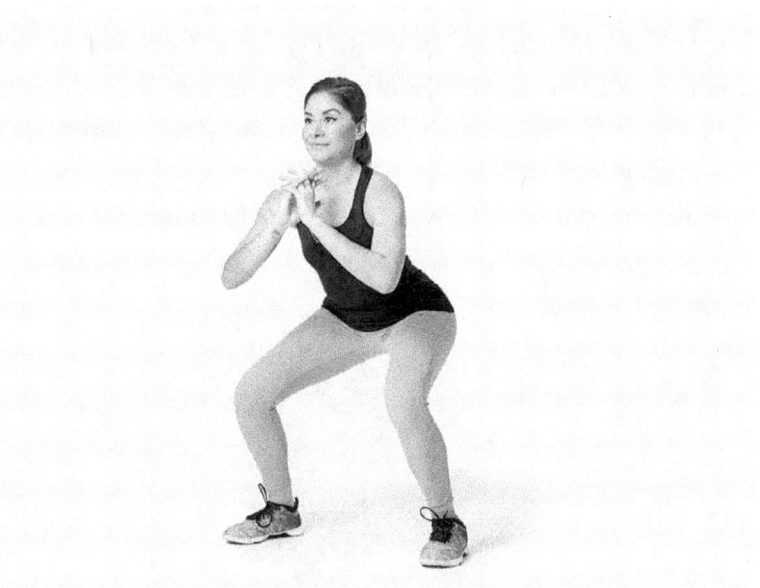

Day 3: Relax

Continue to be mindful of your diet on the day you are taking a break. Do as much unstructured exercise as you can. Go swimming, go for a stroll, or chase your kids around the park.

It is crucial to emphasize that working out does not result in muscle growth if you want to get the most out of your bodybuilding workouts. Instead, during the recovery period following a workout, muscles grow and mend. Because of this, maintaining a healthy diet and getting enough sleep are essential for bodybuilding.

EXERCISE PROGRAMS FOR WOMEN

Day 4: Fundamental

1. Do jumping jacks or jumping rope for ten minutes to warm up. You can also stroll quickly or run in place. Take five more minutes to perform neck rolls, in which you nod affirmatively and then move your head in full circles.

2. Perform 10 shoulder shrugs in 3 sets. Place your feet together and raise your shoulders so they are in line with your ears. Lower them gradually.

3. For a minimum of ten seconds, hold a plank.

4. Perform three sets of ten V-Ups.

5. Take a minimum of ten seconds to hold another plank.

6. Perform 15 Side Bends in 3 sets. Place your feet shoulder-width apart as you stand. Lift the arm on the other side over your head as you bend to one side. Return to the center and raise the second arm above your head while bending the other way.

7. Take a minimum of ten seconds to hold another plank.

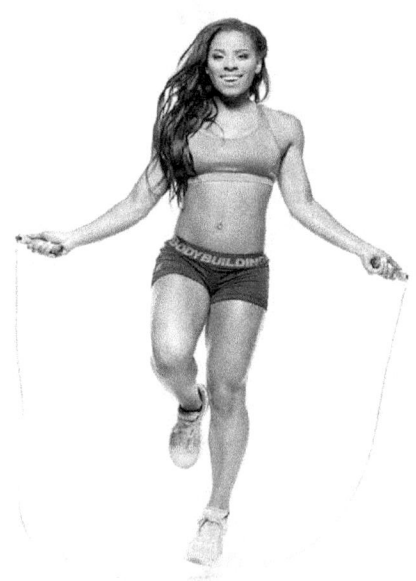

Day 5: Lower Body

1. Start with a quick 10-minute jog or stroll to warm up. Continue

marching and skipping for five more minutes.

2. Perform 12 chair squats in 3 sets. You will perform an identical exercise to a standard squat except that you will be standing in front of a chair. Push yourself back up after lowering yourself to almost the chair.

3. Perform 15 toe raises in 3 sets.

4. Perform 12 side leg lifts in 3 sets. On your right side, lie down on the ground. Extend your legs and use your elbows to support your upper body. Raise and lower your left leg to its maximum height while maintaining your right leg on the ground. Flip and complete the opposite side as well.

5. Perform 10 Side Lunges in 3 sets. Place your hands on your hips and your feet together as you stand. Leap as far to the right as you can without falling, taking a big step. Return to the center position by pushing yourself. Switch to the left side.

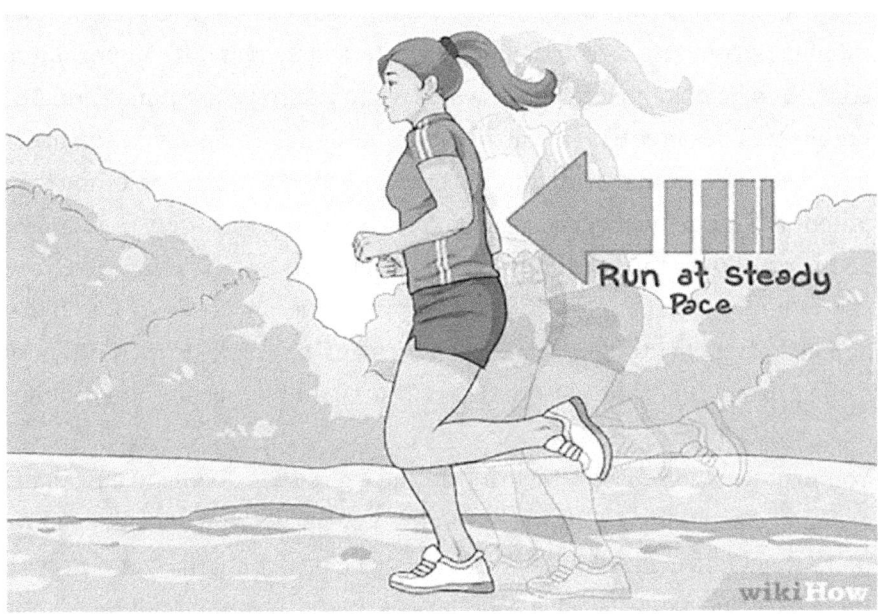

Day 6: Relaxation

It's possible that you're sore, especially after working out your lower body again. Give your body time to relax, and go for a stroll to help your healing muscles get some fresh air.

Day 7: Upper Body and Core

1. Take a ten-minute jog or walk to warm up. Do toe lifts, shoulder rolls, and neck rolls for five minutes.
2. For a minimum of ten seconds, hold a plank.
3. Perform three sets of ten V-Ups.
4. Perform 15 Hip Thrusts in 3 sets.
5. Perform 10 hip lifts in 3 sets.
6. Perform 10 push-ups in 3 sets.

Exercises for Strength Training at Home: Variety

It's critical to avoid growing bored. You'll notice that the repetitions get easier and you can lift heavier weights when using dumbbells, kettlebells, or other weights as your strength and endurance start to increase. It's important to constantly be searching for fresh workouts to add to your strength training regimen. The activities in this book are designed to be easy enough for beginners to begin understanding the physical aspects of their bodies and their potential for personal development. Make sure to do a variety of exercises and learn about other methods to strengthen your body and improve your strength if you start to get bored or the routines become tedious. Recall that although strength training is your primary focus, mild aerobic exercise is also appropriate. It's beneficial to your legs, heart, and general physical health.

You may work on these strength training exercises at home. You can get encouragement for your efforts by joining a gym when you're ready to move on to weight lifting machines. For the time being, familiarize yourself with these basic workouts to lay a solid basis for your training regimen. Some people discover that working out with a friend increases their success rate. If you choose to proceed in this manner, review the strategy and the program to ensure that you are on the right track in light of your goals for improvement and your existing skill level.

3

Nutrition for Bodybuilders: What to Eat

The mechanism by which strength training and exercise result in muscle growth is a key question in bodybuilding. Strength and weight training causes little tearing and damage to your muscle fibers. This triggers the activation of a unique subset of cells called satellite cells, which are found adjacent to the body's muscle cells. Satellite cells that have been activated multiply and merge with the injured muscle fibers to strengthen and mend them. Furthermore, muscle cells are stimulated by satellite cells to produce new proteins. When these things come together, the healed muscles become stronger and thicker than they were before the activity.

It's critical to consider your diet while beginning a strength training program. Your diet will supply your body with energy and the nutrients it needs to grow, repair, and preserve muscle. Eating adequate food to support your optimum physical performance is more important than going on a tight diet and cutting back on meals and calories. Protein is the main component of a diet for bodybuilders since it keeps your metabolism running high and helps you gain muscle mass.

Pay Attention to Protein

The main component of your diet for bodybuilding will be protein. Your cells are fed by protein. It permits all of your tissues—especially your muscle tissue—to proliferate and remain healthy. Protein is also used by your body to make hormones and to keep your blood, skin, and bones healthy. Numerous body processes slow down and suffer when you don't get enough protein in your diet. Your bones could become more brittle, you lose muscle, and your skin and hair start to look lifeless. You need to consume more protein when you start a strength training program because you are not only maintaining but also developing a strong and healthy body.

Foods are the primary source of high-quality protein. Eggs, fish, and lean meats like turkey, beef, and pork are all OK. Nuts and seeds, legumes like beans, and tofu are also sources of protein. Some people use protein bars, powders, and shakes as dietary supplements. This is an excellent method to incorporate the important protein elements into your diet while also giving yourself a boost of energy. To avoid hunger, you should aim to consume as much actual protein as you can. Eat a platter of eggs to start your day. A healthy, high-protein breakfast will provide you with a solid foundation and the energy you need to go through your exercises and the rest of the day.

Incorporating protein into your bodybuilding diet has additional benefits. You won't have to worry about reaching for unhealthy snacks during the day because you'll feel fuller. Because the protein increases your metabolism, it will also aid in fat burning more efficiently. You will experience an increase in energy when your body transforms the protein into glucose. It has also been demonstrated that diets richer in protein and lower in carbs can help with weight loss and improve heart health.

There are lipids in many protein sources as well. Regarding that, don't worry too much. Additionally, your body needs the fat, particularly when you're gaining muscle. Your body is getting what it needs as long as you're eating foods high in healthy fats, such nuts, fish, and oils.

Nutrition before and after exercise

The foods you consume both before and after strength training exercises will have a significant effect on your performance. Eat some high-quality carbohydrates and protein before working out to provide you the energy you need to lift weights and tone your physique. Try some scrambled eggs over a slice of high-fiber toast or some whole-grain oats topped with fruit and nuts if you enjoy working out in the morning. Brown rice or pasta is a fantastic food to eat approximately an hour before you start your strength training if you work out in the afternoon or evening.

You must have some protein after working out because it will aid in muscle recovery. Snack on some fish or grilled chicken. Try a protein shake or a protein bar to nourish and mend your muscles if you're not in the mood for a large meal. Aim to stay hydrated and steer clear of anything high on the glycemic index. These will deplete your energy and make you feel exhausted while doing strength exercise. It is never a good idea to ingest empty carbs, which come from sugars and junk food, particularly right before or right after an exercise session.

Wholesome eating

The majority of bodybuilders who are successful eat a diet rich in protein and healthy carbs. Processed foods that are heavy in added fats, sugar, and salt will only make you gain weight and slow you down. Make sure you're acquiring lean, healthy muscle rather than fat if you do gain weight when bodybuilding. Creating a diet that is nourishing, well-balanced, and appropriate for use in conjunction with a strength training program is one approach to do that.

The best approach is to eat clean. Select sustainable, locally sourced meats and seafood that are high in protein, vitamins, and minerals to help you grow your body. Focus your meals on poultry, turkey, eggs, salmon, and lean beef. Add healthy carbs to that protein, including sweet potatoes, pasta, whole grain bread, and brown rice. To boost your intake of fiber and maintain the health of your body, including some seasonal fruits and leafy green veggies. When it comes to snacking, opt for probiotic foods like yogurt and nuts and seeds.

Eating a clean diet can help you achieve all of your muscle building goals by providing the fuel your body needs to grow muscle. It will be well-fed and primed for action. Twenty delectable and healthful clean eating dishes are included in Chapter 4.

Watch out for fad diets. Even though one of your exercise objectives may be to lose weight, you shouldn't drastically cut back on your caloric consumption. Your body won't be able to grow more muscle and strength if you do that. Consider the kinds of food you're choosing more than how many calories you're consuming. It will be much more important what you consume than how many calories or fat grams are in it.

The diet you need for bodybuilding is important, but exercises come first. The best method to gain muscle is to lift weights on a regular and difficult basis. You'll have to commit to working out more and using weights for longer periods of time. You'll be amazed at the outcomes you can attain when you pair that with the appropriate diet.

4

Recipes for Clean Eating

The majority of eating programs focus on a specific food type, calorie intake, or the proportion of fat to protein in the diet. Eating clean is much easier. The definition of "clean eating" is "eating as naturally as possible." The premise is to consume foods as close to their natural state as possible. This entails choosing uncooked or unrefined meals. Except when you desire them, you are not specifically excluding or including any foods. You don't need to be concerned about protein requirements, calorie counts, or avoiding veggies that are related to nightshades.

Green eggs for breakfast

Produces two portions.
Components:
Four eggs
Two cups of baby spinach leaves
One chopped celery stalk; one sliced zucchini; one diced cup of green bell pepper
One tablespoon of almond milk
One tablespoon of olive oil
To taste, add salt and pepper.

Instructions

1. In a skillet over medium heat, heat the oil. After adding the zucchini, celery, and green pepper, simmer for three minutes.

2. Once the spinach starts to wilt, add it and simmer.

3. Add the almond milk to the eggs after beating them with a fork or whisk. Transfer to a skillet and stir to include all the veggies.

4. Season with pepper and salt.

Data on Nutrition (Per Serving)
229 calories
Weight: 17.8 g; Sat Fat: 5.4 g
6.3 g of carbohydrates
1.9 g of fiber
3.5 g of sugar
13.1 grams of protein

Breakfast Casserole
Four portions Components:
4 chopped and peeled red potatoes
One cup of chopped and peeled eggplant and one cup of chopped and peeled butternut squash
four garlic cloves
One chopped red bell pepper, one chopped green bell pepper, and one sliced ½ red onion
two cups broccoli
Four tsp olive oil
One fresh rosemary sprig
Four new basil leaves
To taste, add salt and pepper.

Instructions:
1. Turn the oven on to 375 degrees Fahrenheit. Stir all the ingredients until they are well blended after adding the olive oil.

2. Bake the vegetables for 40 minutes, or until they are tender and bubbling.

Data on Food (Per Serving)

Calories : 328
Fat : 14.6 g
Sat Fat : 2.1 g
Carbohydrates : 47.5 g
Fiber : 7.6 g
Sugar : 6.9 g
Protein : 6.7 g

Construct Your Own Granola

Produces six servings.
Components:
One cup of almonds
One cup cashews
Half a cup of walnuts
1/4 cup of raisins
One cup of oats
½ cup of coconut, shredded
Half a cup of sunflower seeds
Half a cup of pine nuts
three tsp of cinnamon
Two cups of almond milk

Instructions

1. Using a mixer, thoroughly mix all of the dry ingredients until well incorporated.
2. Divide into four dishes and fill each with ½ cup almond milk.

Nutritional Information (Per Serving)

Calories : 471
Fat : 33.5 g
Sat Fat : 5.5 g

Carbohydrates : 36.4 g
Fiber : 6.8 g
Sugar : 11.9 g
Protein : 13.3 g
Sodium : 55 mg

Smoothie Berry Blast

1 serving is produced. Ingredients:
Half a cup of blueberries
Half a cup of strawberries
1/4 cup raspberries
Half a cup of blackberries
Half a banana
One cup almond milk
½ cup of ice

Instructions:

1. In your blender, combine all the ingredients and blend on high for 30 seconds.

Nutritional Information (Per Serving)

Calories: 240
Fat: 3.9 g
Sat Fat: 0.1 g
Carbohydrates: 51.8 g
Fiber: 12.5 g
Sugar: 30.2 g
Protein: 4.4 g
Sodium: 147 mg

Yield of Carrot

Bread: 8 serves Components:
two cups of almond flour

One tsp baking powder
One tablespoon of seeds from cumin
Add salt to taste.
Three big eggs
Two tsp olive oil
One spoonful of vinegar made from apple cider
Three cups shredded and peeled carrots
One-half teaspoon of freshly peeled and coarsely grated ginger
1/4 cup of raisins

Directions:
1. Preheat the oven to 350 degrees Fahrenheit.
2. Use parchment paper to line a loaf pan.
3. Combine the almond flour, salt, cumin seeds, and baking powder in a big bowl and stir thoroughly.
4. Place the eggs, vinegar, and olive oil in a another bowl and beat until thoroughly mixed.
5. Mix the flour mixture thoroughly after adding the egg mixture.
6. Gently mix in the raisins, carrot, and ginger.
7. Pour the batter into the loaf pan that has been ready.
8. Bake until a toothpick inserted in the center comes out clean, which should take about an hour.

Nutritional Information (Per Serving)
Calories: 133
Fat: 8.9 g
Sat Fat: 1.3 g
Carbohydrates: 10 g
Fiber: 2 g
Sugar: 4.9 g
Protein: 4.5 g

Lunch: 1 serving of Southwest Chicken Wrap

Components:
One tortilla made entirely of whole wheat
¼ cup shredded carrots, diced, and 6 ounces cooked chicken
¼ cup finely chopped red bell pepper and ¼ cup cooked black beans
Two avocado slices
One tsp of dehydrated cilantro
One tsp red pepper flakes
Lime juice from half of a lime

Directions:
1. Place the chicken pieces on the tortilla, then top with avocado, beans, pepper, and carrots.
2. Squeeze the lime over everything after adding the red pepper flakes and cilantro. Make a shawl out of it.

Nutritional Information (Per Serving)
Calories: 565
Fat: 15.9 g
Sat Fat: 3.4 g
Carbohydrates: 47.2 g
Fiber: 13.6 g
Sugar: 5.6 g
Protein: 60 g
Sodium: 260 mg

Yield for the chicken and rice bowl: 1 serving
Components:
½ cup of brown rice, cooked
1/2 cup cooked chicken and 1/2 cup finely chopped tomatoes
Half a cup of cooked corn
1/4 cup black beans, cooked
One lime
To taste, add salt and pepper.

Instructions:

1. Top the brown rice with the chicken, corn, and black beans, and toss to combine.

2. Add salt, pepper, and fresh tomatoes on top. Pour lime juice on top.

Nutritional Information (Per Serving)

Calories: 299
Fat: 3.5 g
Sat Fat: 0.8 g
Carbohydrates: 42.3 g
Fiber: 7.7 g
Sugar: 3.6 g
Protein: 27.7 g

Tuna Salad: Makes two portions.

Components:
Four cups of lettuce
One tuna can in water
One tsp olive oil
One tsp freshly squeezed lemon juice
½ cup chopped sun-dried tomatoes; ½ cup kalamata olives; ½ cup red bell pepper, sliced;
One celery stalk, cut
One tsp of dehydrated oregano

Directions:

1. Wash and pat dry the lettuce, then arrange it like a bed on a dish.

2. Combine the tuna, lemon juice, olive oil, and oregano in a bowl. Incorporate the veggies and blend everything thoroughly.

3. After adding salt and pepper for seasoning, transfer the tuna mixture onto the bed of lettuce.

4. If desired, drizzle with a little additional olive oil.

Nutritional Information (Per Serving)
Calories: 232
Fat: 9.3 g
Sat Fat: 1.6 g
Carbohydrates: 16 g
Fiber: 4.3 g
Sugar: 7.9 g
Protein: 23.5 g
Sodium: 633 mg

Sweet Potatoes with Garlic
1 serving is produced. Ingredients:
Peel and thinly slice one medium sweet potato into round pieces.
One tsp olive oil
To taste, add salt and pepper.
one smashed garlic clove
One tsp carefully cut parsley
¼ cup grated orange peel

Directions:
1. Preheat the oven to 400 degrees Fahrenheit.
2. Combine the sweet potato, oil, salt, and pepper in a bowl.
3. Arrange the potato slices on a sizable baking pan and drizzle with cooking spray. After baking for ten minutes, flip the potato slice and continue baking for an additional ten minutes, or until it turns golden brown.
4. Take out and place the potato slices in a bowl.
5. Combine the parsley, lemon rind, and smashed garlic in a bowl and toss with the sweet potato pieces. Warm up the food.

Nutritional Information (Per Serving)
Calories: 149
Fat: 4.9 g
Sat Fat: 0.7 g

Carbohydrates: 25.2 g
Fiber: 4.1 g
Sugar: 7.4 g
Protein: 2.6 g

Chili with Beans and Turkey Yield: 6 serves
Components:

1. One red onion, one chopped green bell pepper, two pounds of pounded turkey breast, three cloves of garlic, and two tablespoons of olive oil
2. Six fresh tomatoes, diced and seeded, and six ounces of tomato paste
3. One cup of rinsed red kidney beans, one cup of rinsed black beans, one cup of rinsed garbanzo beans, and four tablespoons of ground cumin
4. One tsp finely ground coriander
5. two tsp of chili powder
6. one cup of water
7. Half a tablespoon of salt

Instructions:

1. Cook the turkey in a large soup pot over medium heat for about 10 minutes, or until it is brown. Stir in the chili powder, coriander, and cumin.

2. Take the turkey out of the pot and cover it with olive oil. Saute the bell pepper, onion, and garlic until they are tender.

3. Include the salt and tomatoes. Give the tomatoes ten minutes or so to simmer.

After that, put the beans and tomato paste back into the pot with the meat.

4. Give everything a good stir. Pour water over it. Cook for thirty minutes on low heat with a lid on.

Nutritional Information (Per Serving)

Calories: 745
Fat: 20.4 g
Sat Fat: 4.4 g

Carbohydrates: 76.2 g
Fiber: 20 g
Sugar: 13.7 g
Protein: 67.6 g
Sodium: 758 mg

Munchies

Egg Whites with Deviled Flavor
12 servings are produced.

Ingredients:

6 hardboiled and peeled eggs; ½ cup rinsed capers; ½ cup minced olives; ¼ cup diced red bell pepper

One tablespoon of olive oil

To taste, add salt and pepper.

Instructions:

1. Slice the eggs lengthwise in half, then remove the yolks.
2. Season the egg whites with pepper and salt.
3. Use a fork to mash the capers in a small bowl, then mix in the olives, red pepper, and olive oil. Mix everything together. Fill the spaces on the egg whites with a scoop.

Nutritional Information (Per Serving)

Calories: 49
Fat: 4 g
Sat Fat: 0.9 g
Carbohydrates: 0.9 g
Fiber: 0.3 g
Sugar: 0.3 g
Protein: 2.9 g

Antipasto Kabats

4 servings are produced.

Components:

Two celery stalks, cut into large pieces

One cup of white button mushrooms

One cup of cubed, chilled chicken

cup of hearts of artichokes

One cup of olives

One red pepper, chopped into pieces

One green pepper, chopped into pieces

¼ cup olive oil and two cups of cauliflower florets

One tablespoon of oregano

To taste, add salt and pepper.

Directions:

1. Put everything in a bowl, stir, and drizzle with olive oil.
2. Take a half hour to relax.
3. Put the food on skewers in stacks.

Nutritional Information (Per Serving)

Calories: 244

Fat: 17.6 g

Sat Fat: 2.6 g

Carbohydrates: 11.4 g

Fiber: 4.3 g

Sugar: 4.1 g

Protein: 13.2 g

Nuts and Seeds Roasted

15 servings are produced.

Components:

One cup of almonds

One cup of walnuts

one cup of almonds

one cup of peanuts

½ cup seeds of pumpkin and ¼ cup seeds of sunflower
Half a cup of pine nuts
Two fresh rosemary sprigs
Six freshly cut sage leaves
One-tsp cayenne pepper
One tablespoon of olive oil
To taste, add salt and pepper.

Directions:

1. Warm up an oven to 400 degrees Fahrenheit.

2. Arrange the seeds and nuts on a baking sheet. Add the salt, pepper, olive oil, and cayenne pepper. Add the sage and rosemary.

3. Roast for roughly 20 minutes in the oven.

4. Take out and let cool.

Nutritional Information (Per Serving)

Calories: 228
Fat: 20.9 g
Sat Fat: 2.1 g
Carbohydrates: 6 g
Fiber: 3.1 g
Sugar: 1.1 g
Protein: 8.2 g

Fruit Salad with Cinnamon Yield: 4 servings

Components:
One cup of blueberries and two sliced bananas
1 cup of sliced strawberries and 1 cup of red grapes
One cup of green grapes
One cored, peeled, and diced apple and two cups of cubed watermelon
two tsp freshly squeezed lemon juice
One tablespoon of cinnamon

Instructions:

1. Put all the fruits in a big basin and stir. After adding the lemon juice, toss in all the fruits once more.

2. To allow all the flavors to meld, let the fruits chill for at least thirty minutes.

3. Garnish with the cinnamon and savor.

Nutritional Information (Per Serving)

Calories: 186
Fat: 0.8 g
Sat Fat: 0.2 g
Carbohydrates: 47.5 g
Fiber: 6.2 g
Sugar: 33.1 g
Protein: 2.3 g
Sodium: 6 mg

Fantastic Green Smoothie

1 serving is produced. Ingredients:
Half an avocado
Half a cucumber
one cup of spinach
1 celery stalk and ¼ cup of fresh mint leaves
One tsp finely grated ginger, fresh
one cup of water
½ cup of ice

Instructions:

1. Blend all the ingredients together in a blender until the veggies are well mixed and the ice is broken up.

Data on Nutrition (Per Serving)

Calories: 242

Fat: 20.1 g
Sat Fat: 4.3 g
Carbohydrates: 16.2 g
Fiber: 9.8 g
Sugar: 2.2 g
Protein: 4.3 g
Sodium: 52 mg

Dinner is sour and sweet salmon.

4 servings are produced.

Components:

¾ teaspoon finely chopped fresh ginger root and two tablespoons sliced scallions

1 tablespoon finely chopped garlic

Two tsp olive oil

Half a tsp balsamic vinegar

One tablespoon of honey

½ teaspoon crushed red pepper flakes

Add salt to taste.

Four salmon fillets (6 oz.)

Instructions:

1. Combine all ingredients, excluding salmon fillets, in a large bowl.
2. Include the salmon and liberally brush it with marinade. After about eight hours of marinating, cover and chill, tossing periodically.
3. Set the grill's temperature to medium-high.
4. Oil the grates on the grill. Over the grill grate, place the salmon fillets 5 inches away from the heat source.
5. Grill the salmon fillets for five to ten minutes, turning them once around the halfway point or until they are cooked to your liking.

Nutritional Information (Per Serving)

Calories: 308

Fat: 17.6 g
Sat Fat: 2.5 g
Carbohydrates: 5.5 g
Fiber: 0.2 g
Sugar: 4.5 g
Protein: 33.2 g

Citrus-Fried Shrimp

4 servings are produced.

Components:

One pound of peeled and deveined small to medium shrimp

Two sliced and seeded tomatoes

two limes

¼ cup of newly harvested cilantro

Half a cup of olive oil

To taste, add salt and pepper.

Instructions:

1. Set oven temperature to 375°F. Combine the tomatoes and shrimp in a bowl and toss to coat with olive oil.

2. Transfer to a baking tray and drizzle with lime juice. Add the pepper, salt, and cilantro.

3. Cook until the shrimp turn pink, about 20 minutes.

Nutritional Information (Per Serving)

Calories: 242
Fat: 14 g
Sat Fat: 2.2 g
Carbohydrates: 6 g
Fiber: 1.7 g
Sugar: 2.2 g
Protein: 24.5 g

Recipe for Ginger Steak: 4 serves

Components:
eight smashed garlic cloves

Two tsp finely sliced fresh ginger

One tablespoon of honey

Half a cup of olive oil

To taste, add salt and pepper.

1½ pounds of trimmed flank steak

Instructions:
1. Combine all ingredients, except steak, in a big sealable bag.
2. Add the steak and liberally brush it with marinade.
3. Close the bag and let it marinade for approximately a day in the refrigerator.
4. Take the steak out of the fridge and let it sit at room temperature for about fifteen minutes.
5. Turn up the heat to medium-high and gently grease a grill pan. After removing the steak from the extra marinade, put it in a grill pan.
6. Cook for the desired doneness, 6 to 8 minutes on each side.
7. Take out of the grill pan, let cool for ten minutes, and then slice.
8. Slice into appropriate portions using a sharp knife and serve.

Nutritional Information (Per Serving)
Calories: 471

Fat: 37.9 g

Sat Fat: 1.8 g

Carbohydrates: 7 g

Fiber: 0.3 g

Sugar: 4.4 g

Protein: 24.4 g

Mustard Sauced Chicken
Produced in 1 serving

Components:

A tsp of olive oil

Two deboned, skinned, and halved chicken breasts

One-half tsp salt and one pinch black pepper

Half a cup of chicken stock

One spoonful of mustard dijon

One tsp of butter

One tsp finely chopped parsley

Directions:

1. Preheat the oven to 450 degrees Fahrenheit.

2. Add the oil to the chicken after seasoning it with salt and pepper. Transfer to an ovenproof pan and bake for approximately ten minutes, or until the chicken is nicely browned.

3. After turning, grill the chicken until it is browned on the other side. Take off the chicken from the skillet.

4. Transfer the chicken broth to the pan and let it thicken over medium heat. Stir in the butter, parsley, and mustard.

5. Cover the chicken with the mustard sauce and serve immediately.

Data on Nutrition (Per Serving)

Calories: 414

Fat: 21.4 g

Sat Fat: 5.4 g

Carbohydrates: 1.2 g

Fiber: 0.6 g

Sugar: 0.3 g

Protein: 52.1 g

Sodium: 1251 mg

Curry with Meatballs Yield: 6 servings

Components: Meatballs:

One pound of turkey, ground lean

two beaten eggs

Three tablespoons minced red onion; one-half cup chopped fresh basil leaves; one-half teaspoon finely chopped fresh ginger

four finely chopped garlic cloves

One chopped and seeded jalapeño pepper

One spoonful of paste made from red curry.

One-third tablespoon of fish sauce

Two tsp of coconut oil

Add salt to taste.

Regarding Curry:

One red onion, diced; four minced garlic cloves; one minced jalapeño pepper; ½ teaspoon fresh ginger;

Two tsp red curry paste

One 14-ounce can of coconut milk

two tsp freshly squeezed lime juice

To taste, add salt and pepper.

Instructions:

1. To make the meatballs, combine all the ingredients (except the oil) in a large bowl and stir until thoroughly mixed. Shape the mixture into little balls.

2. Melt coconut oil in a big skillet over medium heat. Cook the meatballs for three to five minutes, or until they are golden brown on all sides. The meatballs should be placed in a bowl.

3. Place the onion and a dash of salt in the same skillet, and cook for three minutes.

4. Sauté the jalapeño, garlic, and ginger for one minute.

5. Include the curry paste and cook for one minute.

6. Include the meatballs and coconut milk, then simmer gently. For roughly ten minutes, simmer while covered on low heat.

7. Garnish with a squeeze of lime juice.

Nutritional Information (Per Serving)
Calories: 370
Fat: 29.5 g
Sat Fat: 20.8 g
Carbohydrates: 9.8 g
Fiber: 2.2 g
Sugar: 3.7 g
Protein: 19 g

5

Beginner's Guide to Strength Training

It's normal to feel eager when you first decide to start a strength training program. Pacing oneself is crucial, though. It is important not to push yourself too hard during your early sessions and risk injury or burnout. These beginner's strength training recommendations can help you focus and dedicate your time to the practice of training without setting unattainable goals for yourself.

First tip: Set Your Own Pace

When you first start out, the only person you have to compete with is yourself, even if you eventually make your way onto the competitive circuit. The idea is to work at your own speed and allow yourself to get better with time. It makes no sense to strive to outshine a workout partner who also does strength training or to measure yourself against someone who have been lifting weights for years.

Maintain your attention on yourself and your goals. Begin cautiously and with as many exercises as you are comfortable with. If you promise yourself that you would lift weights for two hours a day, seven days a week, you will most likely wind up frustrated, sore, and unable to carry on. Make modest, doable goals. Perhaps begin with just two days per week or a small weight. Start out at a slower pace and try to increase it.

Tip 2: Gradually Increase Intensity

Gradually up the intensity once you've found a comfortable and sustainable pace. As your lifting starts to seem easier, go from a 10-pound weight to a 15-pound weight and continuing adding more over time. Follow the same protocol for your repetitions. Begin by lifting eight times, then ten, twelve, and finally fifteen times. You'll discover how your body feels and how much weight your muscles can support. By taking it gradually, you can avoid injuries and avoid giving up if you try to push yourself too hard too quickly. Take your time and have faith in your body. Strength training is a long-term fitness regimen; it's not a race. Every two weeks, up your weight.

Tip 3: Pay Attention to Free Weights

Depending on the gym you go, you may be in awe of the elaborate equipment and sophisticated machinery. But keep in mind that the greatest approach to begin a strength training program is with free weights, which you may use at home as well. You can start with barbells and dumbbells to develop a strong foundation of lean muscle mass, and as you get stronger and seek a more challenging workout, you can progress to the machines. Purchase a set of free weights that come in different sizes and weight ranges so that you can lift weights wherever you are.

Tip 4: Take Breaks

Many newbies want to work out every day since they are so enthusiastic about their intentions. Your muscles will use your rest days to recuperate and mend themselves in preparation for your next workout, but your body needs rest. Separate the muscle parts so that you can work on your arms and chest the following day, and your legs the day after. Strive to maintain a schedule of three or four days a week. This will give you enough of a routine so that you become used to working out every other day without putting too much strain on your body or increasing your chance of injury.

Tip5: Acquire Correct Form

If you are unsure about the proper form or technique for lifting, find a partner who is knowledgeable in these areas or think about hiring a personal trainer. If you pick up poor practices as a novice, it will be difficult for you to break those undesirable habits. This can need you to continue at a lower weight for a while until you can achieve and sustain the proper form. But as you advance, it will be worthwhile.

Tip 6: Put your safety first

Exercise with a companion who can spot you if possible, especially for large lifts. When you begin lifting weight that is greater than you have ever lifted, put on a safety belt and don't be embarrassed to ask for assistance. Experienced bodybuilders can teach beginners a lot, and most people who follow this lifestyle are happy to provide advice and recommendations. Gloves are necessary for some bodybuilders to protect their hands. When working out, exercise caution and take all necessary safety precautions.

Tip 7: Pay Attention to Your Diet

You are aware that diet has a significant role in how well you lift. Thus, avoid junk food, consume a lot of protein, and drink plenty of water before, during, and after exercise. Don't cut calories, and be sure to eat enough to sustain the energy required for your weightlifting activities.

Tip 8: Examine Compound Motions

Start out small and straightforward. Don't make working out too complicated. Do the fundamentals instead. Every week, you should perform shoulder lifts, deadlifts, bench presses, and squats. Concentrate on the fundamentals first, then use your momentum to progress to other lifts that target the specific muscle areas you need to strengthen.

Tip 9: Adhere to Your Schedule

Once you establish a regimen, follow it through. Nothing else will produce the same level of outcomes as consistency. You're getting a decent workout as long as you can train every muscle group once a week and feel that you've pushed yourself without going overboard.

Tip 10: Adopt a Holistic Perspective

Strong physical condition is necessary for strength training. Avoid undermining your plans with drugs, alcohol, and smoking. Aim for a sufficient amount of sleep each night and develop stress management skills. Lifting weights is not enough to develop an exceptional physique. It requires dedication to general well-being.

These ten beginner-friendly strength training suggestions can increase your chances of developing a stronger physique. Take their lead and choose what suits you the most. Your bodybuilding success rate and outcomes will rise as a result.

In summary

For women, strength training has many advantages. It can be customized to meet your exercise level and daily routine. Begin with modest weights and a few repetitions; you'll be shocked at how rapidly your capacity increases. With the help of this book, I hope you can lose weight, burn fat, and develop a toned, slender figure.

I'd like to thank you for reading my book in the end. If you liked the book, kindly take a moment to write a review on Amazon and share your ideas with others. I would be very grateful for that!

6

Beginner's Yoga

Simple Yoga Asanas to Strengthen Your Body,
Reduce Weight, and Calm Your Mind

Overview of Yoga

Yoga is a type of restorative practise that balances the mind, body, and soul. Practitioners can re-establish a connection with both the environment and themselves by using a sequence of breathing and stretching exercises. Yoga disciplines are a collection of mental, spiritual, and physical exercises that originated in ancient India. This well-liked method of physical activity and alleviating tension and anxiety is really one of the six recognized schools of Hindu philosophy. Millions of people all around the world practice and love yoga today. In addition, there are numerous yoga schools, as well as practices and methodologies deeply ingrained in Buddhism, Jainism, and naturally, Hinduism.

The Fundamentals of Yoga

Every yoga practitioner follows their own unique set of values, aspirations, and convictions. Nonetheless, there are a few elements that are shared by all varieties and skill levels of yoga. One of such ideas is to relax. It is not like other forms of exercise where you have to jump, sprint, or lift heavy objects. It will be necessary for you to concentrate on relaxing your body, mind, and soul. It takes effort to ease your muscles into a state of relaxation rather than tension. You'll discover how to teach your body to stay flexible and at ease.

Appropriate breathing is another principle. Yoga, an ascetic and spiritual discipline of Hinduism, teaches practitioners how to control and regulate their breath. The latter is crucial for efficiently connecting with your ideas and expanding your mind's eye, as well as for lowering daily stress, anxiety, and tension.

Yoga also emphasizes nutrition, which is one of the main reasons it's so effective for weight loss. You'll be aware of the fuel you're giving your body when you work to maintain the harmony between your life and spirit. The idea is to feed your body and mind fresh, healthful foods. For the serious practice of yoga, you need a light and powerful body, and eating well can help you get there faster. And finally, yoga emphasizes meditation. This method reunites the body and soul as a single, harmonious whole while clearing the mind of mental clutter.

A Synopsis of Yoga's Past

Although there is disagreement on the actual beginnings of yoga, the majority of practitioners give India around 3000 B.C. credit. This is the area in the Indus Valley where sculptures carved into stone depict individuals doing yoga. These pictures show yoga as it was originally practiced, centuries before any modern, current, or social improvements. One of the most important ways to ensure harmony between the heart and soul was and still is through yoga. The goal of every "yogi" (practitioner, disciple, teacher, or guru) is to become enlightened by the divine. This is basically the recognition of a higher force, which to some may be God and to others nature and the heavens.

The Eight-Limbed Yoga Path

Patanjali's Yoga Sutra contains the eight limbs of yoga. Ashtanga is the name of these fundamental principles, which are meant to assist practitioners in living meaningful and purposeful lives. These legs provide guidance on morality, self-control, and appropriate ethics as a route to heavenly illumination. In a similar vein, they support us in recognizing and addressing the spiritual facets of our nature and existence in addition to enhancing our longevity and general health. These are Patanjali's eight limbs of yoga:

Yama

Yama is the name of the first limb in yoga. This discipline aids in helping us pay attention to our actions as well as appropriate behavior in daily life. In a same vein, it imparts moral principles and integrity to us. Yamas, also referred to as the Golden Rule, are intended to be universal norms. The adage "do unto others as you would have them do unto you" obviously applies here. As an illustration, respect for others breeds respect for oneself.

Niyama

We refer to the second limb as niyama. This limb is focused on spiritual observances and self-discipline. For instance, participating in religious activities and saying the grace before meals are crucial for maintaining one's spiritual health. Comparably, going on solo walks or regular meditations help you connect with your inner self and discover your purpose for being on Earth.

Asana

We refer to the third limb as asanas. These are the poses practiced in yoga, which regards the body as the spirit's temple. Asanas, according to yogis, enhance our general health, discipline, attention, and spiritual development. Additionally, asanas are essential in providing us with the inner strength to meditate and focus for harmony, tranquility, and happiness on the inside as well as the outside.

Yamada

We refer to the fourth limb as pranayama. To master and manage our respiratory performance and function, this is basically breath control. Along with learning how healthy breathing may enhance our minds and emotions, we also learn about the relationship between breath and life. Yoga practitioners believe that pranayama, which translates to "life force extension," restores and renews the mind, body, and soul/spirit. You can practice this technique alone or in conjunction with your regular yoga practice.

The Pratyahara

Pratyahara is the name of the fifth branch of yoga. This basically implies removing oneself from the outer world, its surroundings, and its stimulation. Pratyahara, a type of sensory transcendence, is a deliberate attempt to achieve a degree of separation from our senses. We focus our entire attention inside when we employ this strategy. This enables us to take a step back from daily life and effectively examine ourselves from the inside out. We also learn about our habits and urges, which can be detrimental to our general health, wellbeing, and quality of life.

Dharana

The sixth limb of yoga is called dharana. It is crucial to understand that every yoga limb or level gets us ready for the one after it. Keeping this in mind, pratyahara comes before dharana, or concentration. We may control the diversions, straying thoughts, and other stimuli that bother our regular minds and thoughts by using this limb. This type of focus also establishes the guidelines for appropriate meditation practices. Dharana teaches us how to strengthen our focus skills while slowing down the thought process. By doing this, we are able to take charge of our thoughts and brains rather than letting them rule us. Once you have mastered this technique, you will enter a daily state of continuous meditation on its own.

Dhyana

The seventh limb of yoga, dhyana, is focused on maintaining an unbroken stream of attention. While dharana is known as concentration, dhyana is known as meditation. There is a thin line between these limbs, even though these stages are both interwoven. Dharana, for instance, is used to achieve one-pointed attention, whereas dhyana is awareness without focus. When you are in a dhyana state, your mind is calm and you have few or no thoughts.

At this point, your strength and endurance also improve. But yoga is not about perfection per se; rather, it is about discipline, daily instruction, and following. This implies that nothing is ever insurmountable, but if you are unable to accomplish a goal, it's acceptable to go on with your life. Regardless of your skill level or stage, yoga offers mental and physical health advantages at every level.

Samadhi

Samadhi is the eighth and last stage, or limb, in yoga. In this ecstasy-like condition that occurs naturally, the practitioner feels a connection to the Divine. This is also regarded as the final state of meditation, where your attention and point of view have become one with the self. Recall that yoga can only be experienced; it cannot be "mastered" per se. This holds true for every stage at which spiritual awareness could manifest.

Yoga Styles

There are many various styles of yoga, and the best outcomes will come from selecting a style that is appropriate for your skill level and aspirations. Hatha yoga is an excellent way for newcomers to experience yoga. Try out this gentle style of breathing and stretching if you're new to yoga or have never done it before. It will feel calming and rejuvenating.

Vinyasa yoga is another well-liked kind of yoga. This is particularly beneficial for because you are always moving, those who are trying to lose weight from one position to another and one pose to another. As a result, you receive a little combine a cardio exercise routine with your yoga practice. Up to seven can be burned. calories per minute by combining various floor exercises, lunges, and standing positions.

You can increase your flexibility and lose weight by practicing Bikram yoga. It's utilized in "hot yoga" workouts, which take place in studios that are Very warm. Sweating out one's body is considered beneficial by practitioners. contaminants and poisons when practicing yoga.

Yoga's advantages

Yoga has numerous advantages for your mental, emotional, and physical well-being. It can help you feel lighter, stronger, and younger. Exercise not only tones your body, burns calories, and improves your appearance, but it also provides you with a comprehensive approach to physical fitness and overall wellbeing. Yoga teaches your body to be adaptable, open, and in harmony with your heart and intellect. It's excellent for folks who want to concentrate on breathing, stretching, and reaching the elusive condition of inner serenity. It can be added to an existing fitness regimen.

Yoga's Benefits for Losing Weight: Body

Few people are aware of how effective yoga can be as a calorie burner. It won't make you leap about and perspire as cross-training, basketball, or running does. When you practice yoga for thirty or sixty minutes, you do, in fact, consistently burn calories. With poses and stances found in Hatha yoga, even a basic yoga practice can help you burn about 300 calories in an hour. You can burn even more if you up the ante and practice a more strenuous style of yoga, like Vinyasa or Ashtanga. Any form of movement offers the chance to burn calories.

Another important advantage of yoga for weight loss is increasing body awareness. You have to pay attention to what your body is doing and how you are moving in every stance and position. You will have a keen awareness of the way your body functions as a whole and a deep sense of connection with every muscle and limb.

One of the main benefits of yoga is increased flexibility. Your range of motion and balance will improve as a result of all the stretching you perform. You'll see an improvement in your movement and breathing patterns in addition to your posture. Although it may not seem like it would have a significant effect on weight loss, it does. Your physical fitness level automatically rises when you can move more easily. This helps you stay active and burn fat off your body. Better fitness equates to more flexibility. You'll discover that even while you're completing basic tasks, you feel better and look better in your clothes.

Yoga's Benefits for Losing Weight: Mind

Yoga combines mental and emotional well-being with physical conditioning. Positive thinking is crucial to weight loss success. By including a consistent yoga practice into your weight loss plan, you are teaching your mind to use optimism and intention as powerful tools. You can use this time to picture yourself as healthier, stronger, and thinner as you stretch and hold poses. Being in an expectant state will allow weight loss to come to you organically. Yoga will assist you in connecting with your intention and using it to your advantage. Your mind is a potent tool in the weight reduction war.

Stress management is just as important to weight management as giving up junk food and upping physical activity. Anxiety and overwhelm can cause an emotional imbalance that can lead to negative behaviors. When tension begins to overwhelm your body and mind, yoga helps you stay composed and teaches you how to guide yourself back to that level of calm. That awareness will help you stay optimistic and in balance.

Yoga is an empowering, life-changing practice. Whether you're starting out or enhancing an existing practice, you'll notice an immediate improvement in your appearance and well-being.

7

Beginner's Two-Week Yoga Training Plan:

Week One

Yoga may be practiced practically anyplace, doesn't require any special equipment, and doesn't require any special ability to begin. For those who want to practice at home or are new to the activity, these factors make it a great choice. While there aren't many strict rules about what to wear for yoga, it's usually a good idea to wear yoga pants, leggings, or shorts, along with a top that fits comfortably but not too tight. In addition, you should practice on a mat or blanket as well as barefoot.

You will learn and practice new, basic yoga postures every day for two weeks with this two-week training plan. On Sundays, you will review all of the poses you have learned so far. You will learn the starting and finishing poses for every yoga session on the first day.

Monday of the first week: Corpse and Easy Pose

The Easy stance is the first stance that needs to be learned. Each session will start with you in this stance.

1. Take a seat and extend your legs in front of you, crossing them at the shins.

2. Bend your legs inward toward yourself, putting each foot beneath the knee of the person on the other side.

3. Place your hands, palms up or down, on your knees.
4. Sit up straight and distribute your weight equally over your hip bones.
5. Lengthen your spine and align your head, neck, and spine.
6. With your chest out, lower and back your shoulders.
7. Take deep breaths and maintain this stance for fifteen minutes.

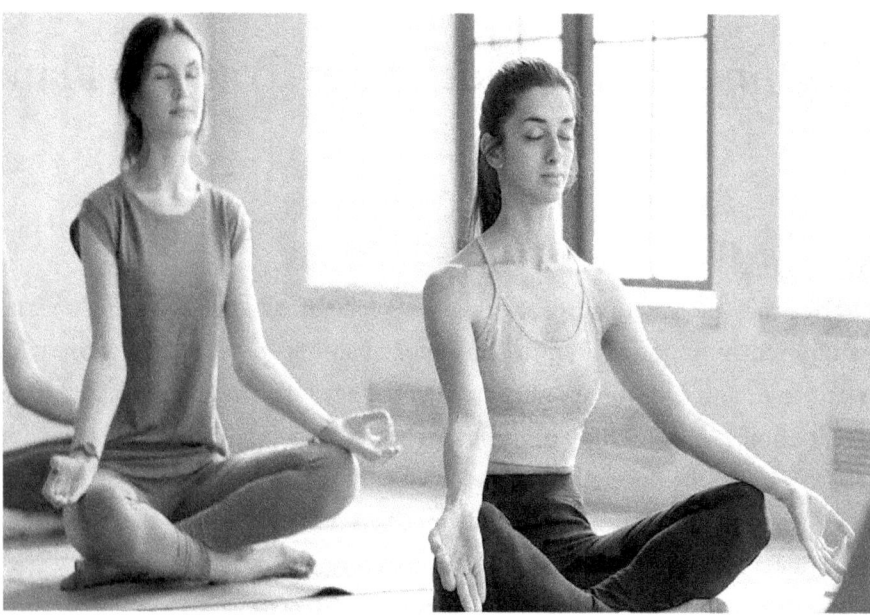

The Corpse stance is the second stance you should learn. You will conclude each session in this stance, which is regarded as the most crucial to learn.

BEGINNER'S TWO-WEEK YOGA TRAINING PLAN:

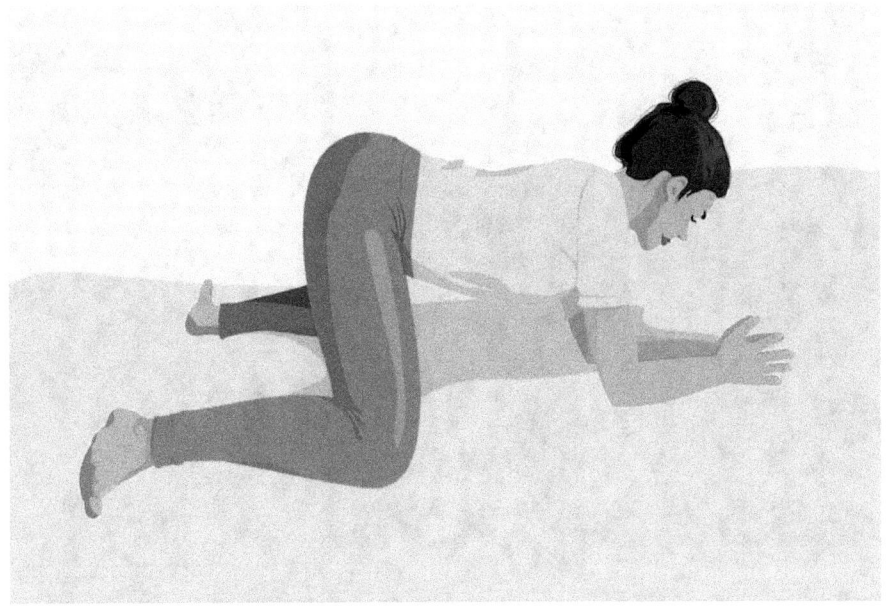

1. While lying on your back, place your arms, palms up, six inches from your sides.

2. Take a natural breath.

3. Shut your eyes and start to deliberately release every muscle in your body, starting from your head and ending at your toes.

4. Maintain this position for a maximum of fifteen minutes.

Tuesday: Forward Bend

1. Start in the easy pose and stay there for five minutes.

2. Place your feet hip-width apart and stand tall to begin the Mountain Pose.

3. Maintain a balanced weight and relaxed shoulders while keeping your arms by your sides.

4. Breathe deeply, then raise your hands and extend your fingers upwards.

5. Hold while taking deep breaths for up to a minute.

6. Return to the initial position, keeping your hands by your sides, and perform the stretch multiple times.

7. Spend the final five minutes in corpse pose.

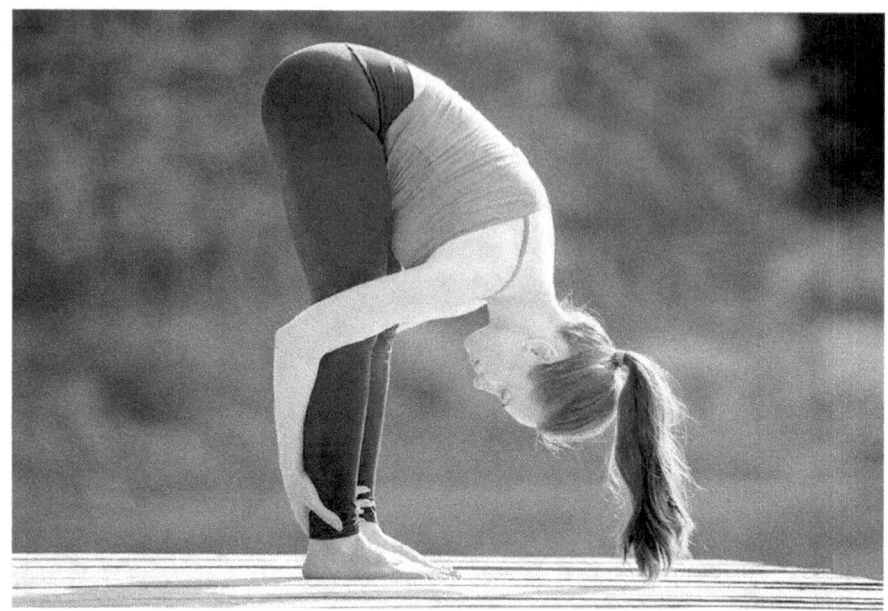

Wednesday: Eagle Salute

1. Start in the easy pose and stay there for five minutes.
2. Place your feet three to four feet apart to begin the Warrior Pose.
3. With your left foot slightly inward, rotate your right foot ninety degrees.
4. Extend your body out to your sides, palms down, while maintaining a comfortable stance at your hips and shoulders.
5. Maintain your right knee over your ankle while bending it to a 90-degree angle.
6. Maintain the stance for a minute by gazing out over your right hand.
7. Change sides and continue as many times as desired.

BEGINNER'S TWO-WEEK YOGA TRAINING PLAN:

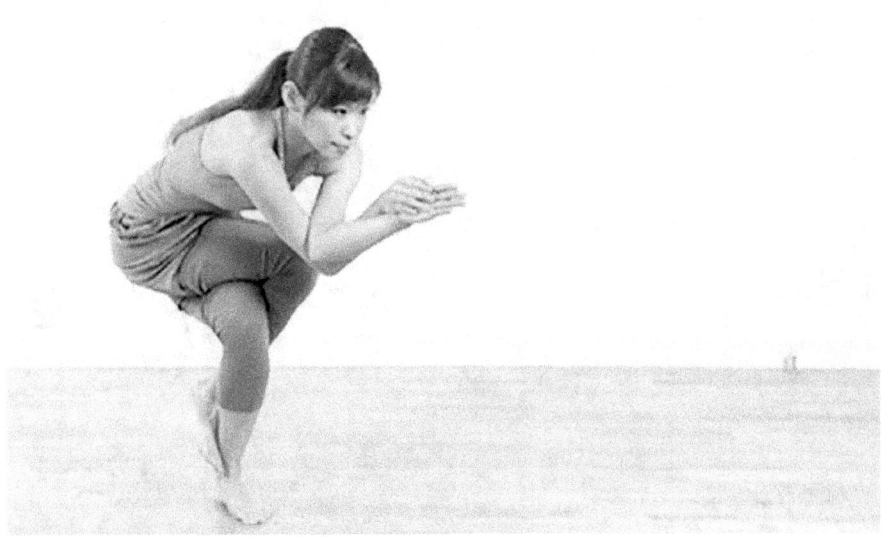

8. Spend the final five minutes in corpse pose.

Thursday: Inverted Dog

1. Start in the easy pose and stay there for five minutes.

2. On your hands and knees on the floor, begin Downward Dog.

3. Place your knees beneath your hips and your hands beneath your shoulders.

4. Spread your fingers wide and place your palms flat on the ground as you slowly stroll your hands forward.

5. Toes should be curled under, hips should be raised, and knees should be slightly bent. Your body should resemble an inverted V.

6. Take three deep breaths into this stance, holding it. You are free to repeat the entire process as often as you wish.

7. Spend the final five minutes in corpse pose.

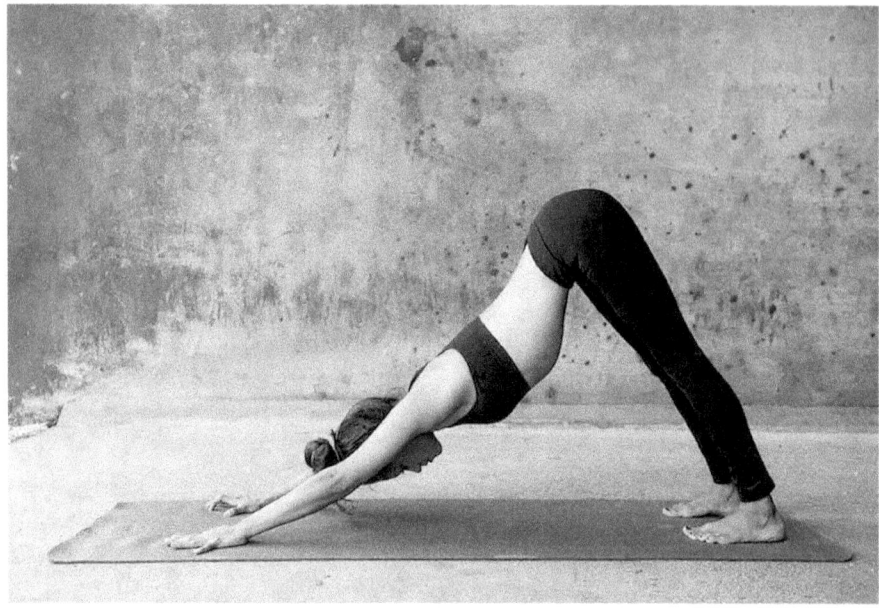

Friday: Standing in a tree

1. Start in the easy pose and stay there for five minutes.

2. With your arms by your sides, stand tall and straight to begin the Tree Pose.

3. Maintaining your forward hip position, transfer your weight to your left leg and insert the tip of your foot into your left thigh.

4. After finding your balance, raise your hands in front of you and place your palms together in the prayer posture.

5. Taking a deep breath, raise your arms above your shoulders, keeping your palms apart and facing each other. Hold this position for 30 seconds.

BEGINNER'S TWO-WEEK YOGA TRAINING PLAN:

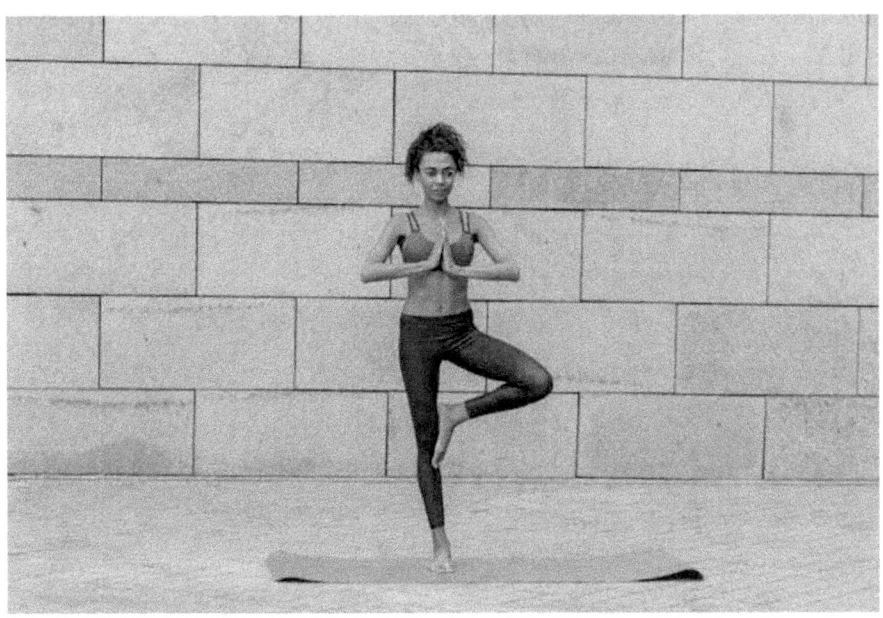

6. Drop your arms, then do the same on the other side.

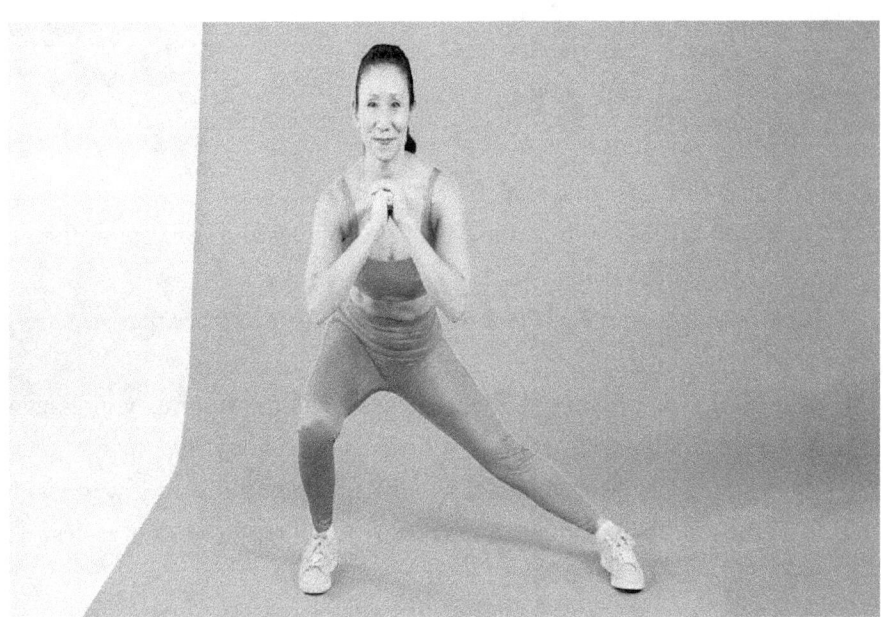

7. Repeat as many times as you desire, switching between the left and right sides.

8. Spend the final five minutes in corpse pose.

Bridge Pose on Saturday

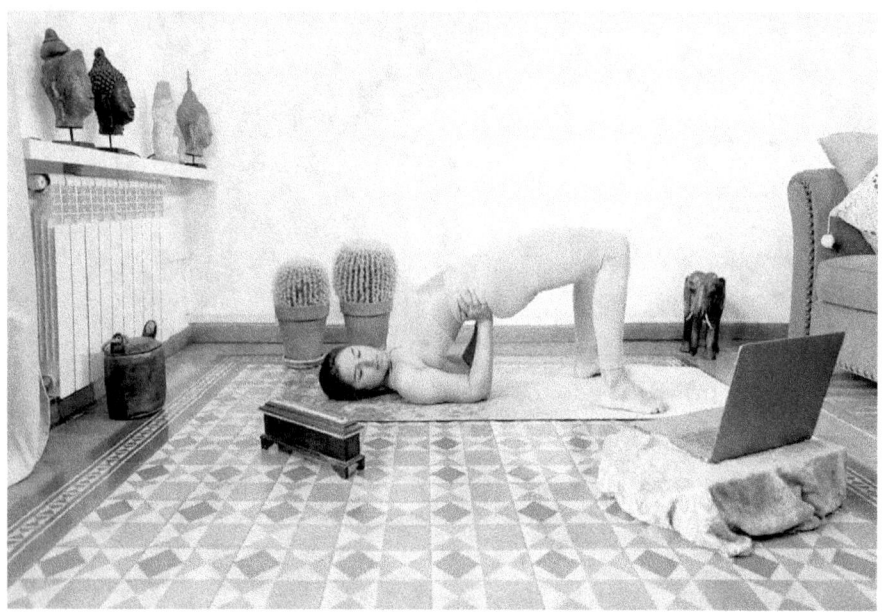

1. Start in the easy pose and stay there for five minutes.

2. Laying on the floor with your arms at your sides and your palms flat on the ground, begin the Bridge Pose.

3. Plant both feet on the ground, bend your knees, and place them squarely over your heels.

4. Lift your hips till your thighs are parallel to the floor as you exhale, pressing your feet into the ground.

5. Press your arms down and place your hands beneath your lower back.

6. Hold the stance for a minute, then release it and repeat as often as desired.

7. Spend the final five minutes in corpse pose.

Sunday: Review of Week One and Child's Pose

For one minute, begin in Easy Pose. Then, hold each of the following poses for one minute: Mountain, Warrior, Downward Dog, Tree, and Bridge. Make sure to perform each stance for Warrior and Tree for one minute on the right and left sides. Following the review, move on to Sunday's new pose, Child Pose, and conclude with Corpse Pose as usual.

Child's Position

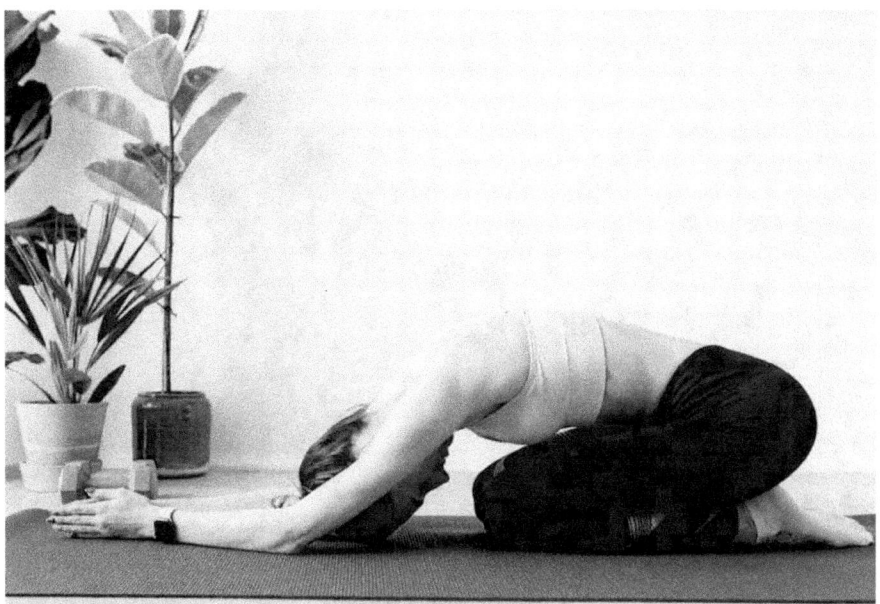

1. Sit up straight on your heels to begin Child's Pose after reviewing the first week.

2. Lean forward so that your forehead is flat on the ground in front of you.

3. Stretch your arms straight out in front of you and get your chest as close to your knees as is comfortable.

4. Press your palms firmly into the earth.

5. Take a deep breath, hold this position for one minute, and then repeat as many times as you'd like.

6. Spend a minute in corpse pose to finish.

8

Beginner's Two-Week Yoga Training Plan: Week Two

You will learn one new pose every day for the second week, and at the end of the week, you will review every stance you learned during the second week.

Monday: Pose in Triangle

EXERCISE PROGRAMS FOR WOMEN

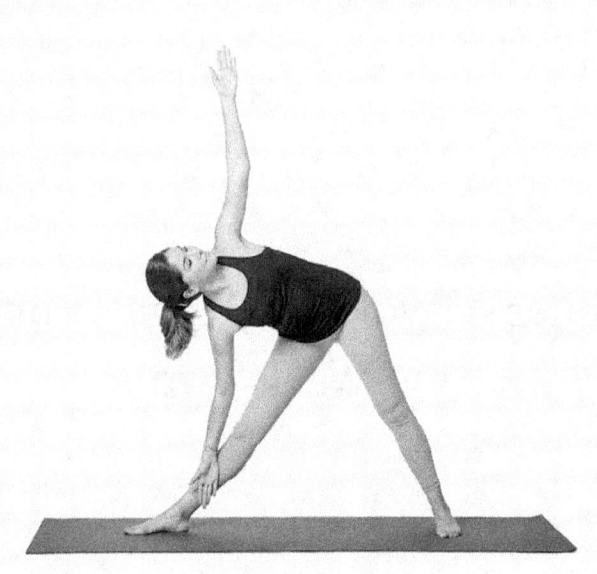

1. Start in the easy pose and stay there for five minutes.

2. To begin Triangle Pose, stand upright with your feet shoulder-width apart and your arms out to the sides.

3. Extend your left foot to a 45-degree angle and your right foot to a 90-degree angle.

4. While maintaining a straight posture, touch your right hand to your right foot.

5. Extend your left hand toward the sky, looking past it, and hold the position for five breaths.

6. Continue on the other side.

7. Repeat as many times as you desire, switching between the left and right sides.

8. Spend the final five minutes in corpse pose.

Tuesday: Dog facing upward

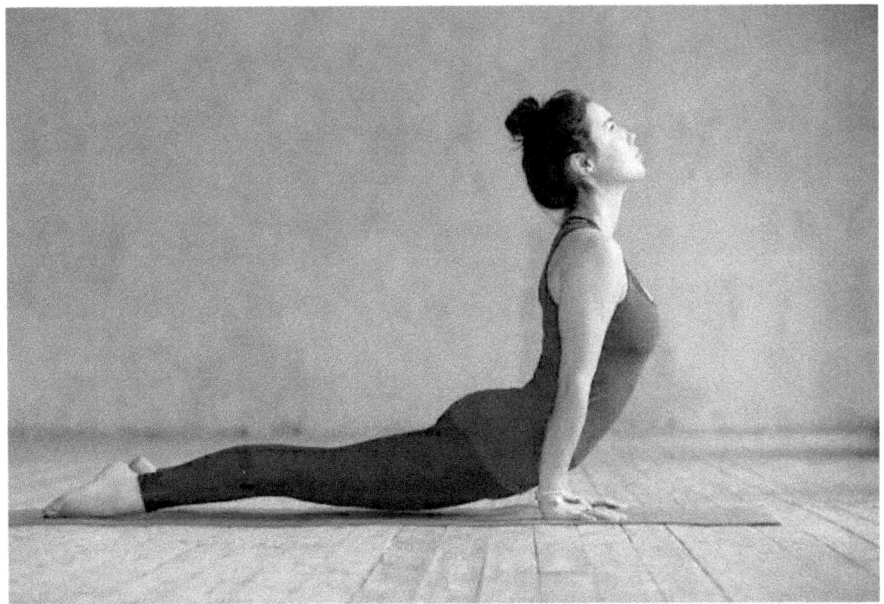

1. Start in the easy pose and stay there for five minutes.
2. Lay face down on the floor to begin the Upward Facing Dog pose.
3. Immediately beneath your shoulders, place your hands flat on the floor, palms down.
4. Stretch your legs out from behind you while maintaining your toes on the ground.
5. Tighten your pelvic floor and tuck your hips down while compressing your buttocks.
6. Keeping your hips on the floor, press your hands into the earth and lift your chest off the surface.
7. Hold for a minute, then release tension and repeat as often as desired.
8. Spend the final five minutes in corpse pose.

Wednesday: In a chair, twist

EXERCISE PROGRAMS FOR WOMEN

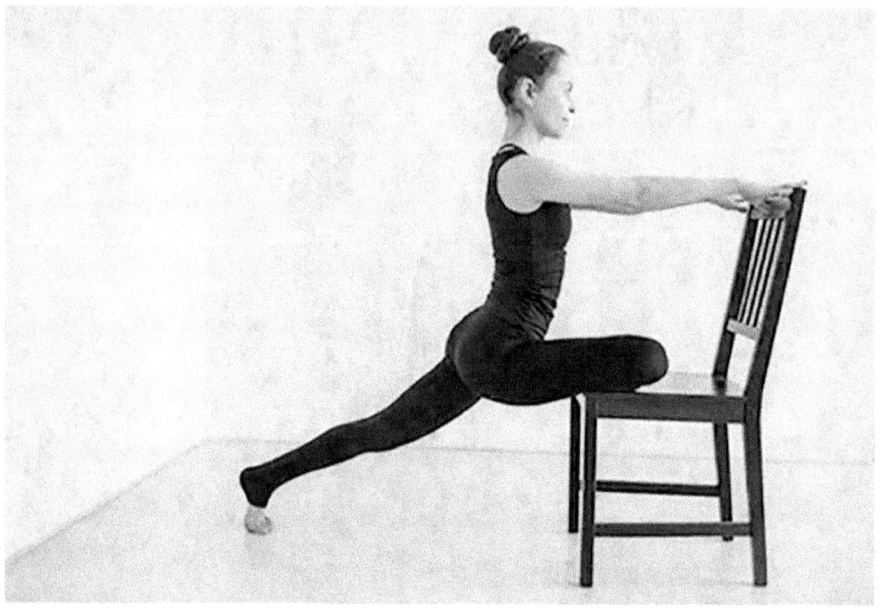

1. Start in the easy pose and stay there for five minutes.

2. To begin the Seated Twist, sit on the floor and extend your legs straight in front of you.

3. Place your right foot outside of your left thigh and over it.

4. Bend your left knee while pointing your right knee up toward the sky.

5. Slide your left elbow to the outside of your right knee while maintaining your right hand on the floor for support.

6. With your buttocks on the floor on both sides, twist to the right as far as feels comfortable starting from your abdomen.

7. Hold for a maximum of 60 seconds.

8. Flip to the other side.

9. Repeat as many times as you desire, switching between the left and right sides.

10. Spend the final five minutes in corpse pose.

Thursday: Pose with pigeons

BEGINNER'S TWO-WEEK YOGA TRAINING PLAN: WEEK TWO

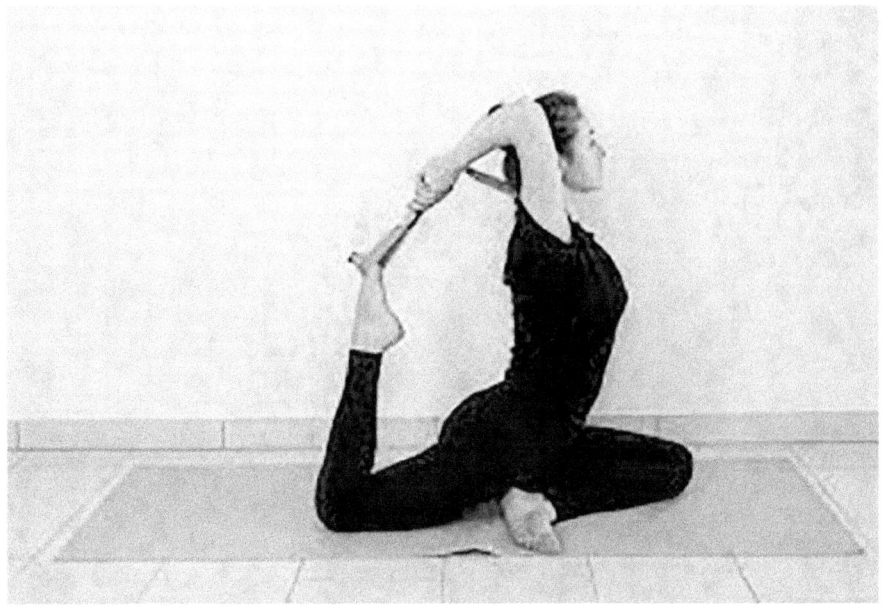

1. Start in the easy pose and stay there for five minutes.
2. Place your hands directly beneath your shoulders, palms down, to begin Pigeon Pose.
3. Lower your left knee to the ground in close proximity to your shoulder. Place your left heel next to your right hip.
4. Lift your chest and sit back by pressing your hands into the ground.
5. Maintain this position for a maximum of one minute.
6. Flip to the other side.
7. Repeat as many times as you desire, switching between the left and right sides.
8. Spend the final five minutes in corpse pose.

Friday: Pose like a dolphin

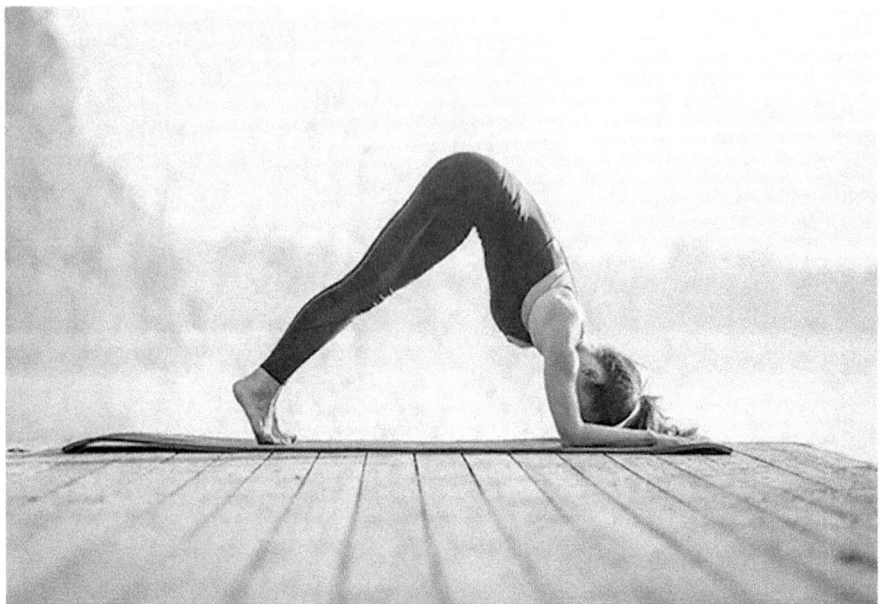

1. Start in the easy pose and stay there for five minutes.
2. From Downward Dog Pose, transition into Dolphin Pose.
3. Lower your forearms to the floor while in the downward dog position.
4. Maintaining shoulder-width hands, spread your fingers widely.
5. Place your forehead on the ground, take a deep breath, and hold the position for a minute.
6. Spend the final five minutes in corpse pose.

Half Wheel Pose on Saturday

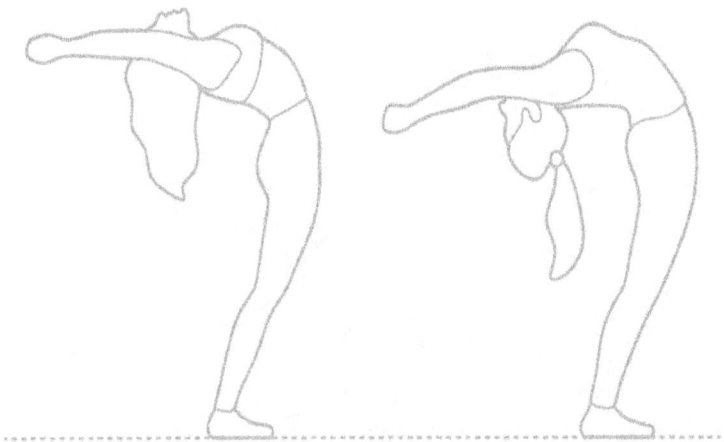

1. Start in the easy pose and stay there for five minutes.
2. Enter Bridge Pose to begin Half Wheel Pose.
3. In the bridge position, raise your hips as high as you can, then shift your weight off your heels and only onto your toes.
4. Keep your hands flat and your arms flat on the ground. As long as a minute, maintain this posture.
5. Spend the final five minutes in corpse pose.

Sunday: Boat Pose and Review of Week Two

After holding each pose for one minute, alternate between Easy Pose and Triangle Pose, Upward Facing Dog, Seated Twist, Pigeon Pose, Dolphin Pose, and Half Wheel Pose. Make sure to perform the Triangle, Seated Twist, and Pigeon poses for one minute on both the right and left sides. Following the review, proceed to the new pose for Sunday, Boat Pose, and finish in Corpse Pose as usual.

Boat Position

EXERCISE PROGRAMS FOR WOMEN

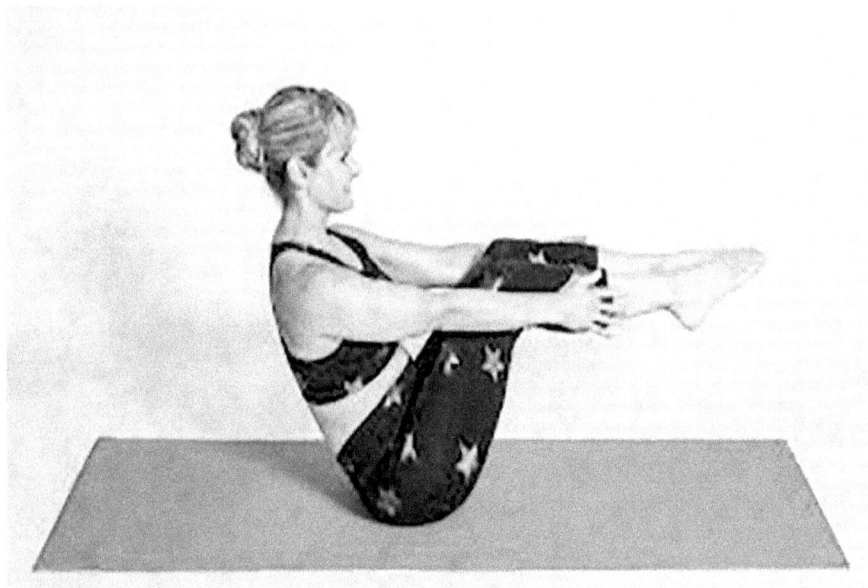

1. Begin in Boat Pose by sitting on the floor with your legs extended in front of you following the Week 2 Review.
2. Keep your legs straight and squeeze them together.
3. To maintain balance, keep your arms parallel to your body and slant your back slightly as you raise your legs off the ground to form a V with your torso.
4. Maintain the stance for as long as you can, noticing the muscles in your thighs and stomach working to hold you still.
5. Let go and repeat the stance as often as you'd like.
6. Spend a minute in corpse pose to finish.

You can repeat this training plan every two weeks after the second week, or you can make up your own by arranging the positions that work best for you.

9

Advice for Newbies to Yoga

Yoga is an exciting new endeavor. You should be willing to work at your own pace and maintain an open mind if you have never done this before and are unsure of what to anticipate. It's not necessary for you to learn the trickiest poses and positions straight away. This chapter contains some advice that will equip you with the resources and self-assurance you need to get going. The most crucial piece of advice is to persevere. You're making a long-term, wise decision when you commit to practicing yoga as a way to reduce weight and improve your health. Yoga is not a fitness fad or trend. You'll discover quickly that it's a way of life.

How to Proceed

Making friends is one of the most crucial things you can do. Yoga is a very beneficial exercise when done alone, but when you have a partner, it becomes an activity you look forward to for both social and health reasons. Join a class that meets at least once a week if you can't find somebody to practice yoga with. Many like-minded individuals who are eager to assist you in developing your yoga practice will come across your path.

Creating a room in your home for yoga is another important "to do". It's not necessary to have a yoga studio set up with mirrors on every wall and a stack of mats. Even if your lessons are in a studio or gym, having a small space where you can stretch when you're tense will assist. Pay attention to the mental and emotional aspects of yoga in addition to the physical.

In class and on your own, you'll be moving and stretching a lot. Thus, set aside the time required to meditate, focus on your breathing, engage in visualization and positive thinking. Your daily life should incorporate your yoga practice.

Things Not to Do

Avoid evaluating yourself against others. Even the easiest pose in yoga, Mountain Pose, can be difficult to hold when you're just starting out. It's alright. That one posture might take up your whole day, or even a week. You are not in a race against anyone, and there is no deadline. Take inspiration and motivation from others around you who have achieved more, but resist the urge to give in to emotions of inferiority or insecurity.

Don't overthink things. Trying to do too much too soon might lead to burnout. Exercise for 30 or 60 minutes three times a week at first, then gradually increase the frequency as your body becomes used to the new demands you're placing on it.

Never let negativity to get in your way. If your well-meaning friends try to convince you that practicing yoga won't help you lose weight, accept their advice and carry on. To improve your health and reduce your waist size, you don't need to run marathons or spend hours lifting weights.

Investments That Are Required

Start constructing a library. Purchase DVDs and videos, and read books and magazines. Purchase some CDs and read through yoga blogs. These will not only keep you informed and educated, but they will also inspire you.

Invest in a quality mat. Your yoga mat will determine whether or not your class is uncomfortable or enjoyable. Try out a couple yoga mats before making a purchase; there are plenty of them available. Find out what and why other people appreciate certain mats by asking them about their usage of them. Invest in yoga attire that fits comfortably, wicks away moisture, and lets you breathe.

Fitted tops, shorts, and pants will let your body to flow naturally into your positions. But anything too tight will feel awkward.

Conscientious Consumption

It's crucial to obtain plenty of sleep before starting a yoga practice. Both your body and mind require rest and renewal. Maintaining your body's strength and alignment with the positive energy flow you're attempting to create also greatly depends on what you eat. You are aware of the fundamentals of weight loss: consume foods that will strengthen rather than deplete you and burn more calories than you take in. You should establish a few basic eating guidelines for yourself. These tips will not only help you shed pounds, but they will also improve your body's flexibility for yoga.

Get rid of the clutter. Simply refuse the packaged goods, sugar-filled foods, fast food, and processed foods that are high in fat, sodium, and sugar. Steer clear of them. You can practice the technique of bringing your mind, body, and soul into balance by doing yoga. Junk eating will make you worse off.

Instead, pay attention to what's in season, local, and fresh. When you're hungry, load up on fruits and veggies. A handful of ripe berries in the spring, or a clementine orange in the fall, should be your initial goal. Make frequent trips to the farmer's market in your community.

You'll get the energy you need for yoga by consuming lean protein. Cook using fish that is high in omegas, such as salmon and sardines, eggs, almonds, and skinless chicken breasts. You'll need to obtain your protein from other foods if you're a vegetarian, such as beans and lentils, tofu, and robust veggies like squash, eggplant, and mushrooms.

In summary

You can get a good start to your yoga practice with this book. Maintain a high degree of energy and excitement and get enthused about all the fascinating things yoga can teach you about your body and health. This isn't your typical exercise regimen. It changes the way you think about everything, including eating and weight loss, by reaching into your spirit. Stay open-minded and physically flexible, and be prepared to go wherever this path leads you. I'd like to thank you for reading my book in the end. If you liked the book, kindly take a moment to write a review on Amazon and share your ideas with others. I would be very grateful for that!

www.ingramcontent.com/pod-product-compliance
Lightning Source LLC
LaVergne TN
LVHW020431080526
838202LV00055B/5133